FIERCE BLESSING

BY THE AUTHORS

Adult Nonfiction:

Fierce Blessing

Young Adult & Children's Fiction:

Night Of The Falling Stars
The Invisible Kid And Dr. Poof's Magic Soap
The Invisible Kid And The Killer Cat
The Invisible Kid And The Intergalactic RV

FIERCE BLESSING

A Journey Into Alzheimer's,
Compassion, and the Joy of Being

Wayne and Terry Baltz

PRAIRIE DIVIDE PRODUCTIONS
Red Feather Lakes, Colorado

Prairie Divide Productions
P.O. Box 129
Red Feather Lakes, CO 80545
888-288-4841
http://www.fierceblessing.com

Cover design & photograph copyright © 2003 by Gary Raham

This book is a memoir. It portrays actual events. However, in order to preserve the privacy of those involved, the names, locations, times, and other details have been changed or otherwise disguised and some characters mentioned in this book are composites. Since names, places, and other details have been disguised or changed, with the exception of the names of the authors and the members of their family, the similarity of the name of any character or place in this book to any actual person or place is merely coincidental.

Due to limitations of space, permissions and acknowledgments of copyrighted material are included on the facing page and should be considered to be part of this copyright page.

The text of this book is set in Perpetua.
Printed in the United States of America on acid-free, recycled paper.

Library of Congress Control Number: 2002113056

ISBN   1-884610-71-4

Special quantity discounts are available on bulk purchases of this book for promotions, educational purposes, subscription incentives, or fund raising. Please visit http://www.fierceblessing.com or call 888-288-4841 (ask for Special Sales).

PERMISSIONS & ACKNOWLEDGMENTS

For
HELEN

— *Prologue* —

The call comes in the middle of the night. Every cell in my body knows I cannot answer. I wrestle the phone off the night stand.

"Wayne," I say, and pass it to him beside me in the bed. He fumbles with the headset, hoists it clumsily to his cheek.

"Hello?" His voice is aged and deepened by sleep.

My fingers trace the cord that stretches across my chest in the silent dark.

It's Lilith. I know that.

— 1 —

The world is but a bridge, build no house upon it.
Life is but an hour, spend it in devotion.
All the rest is the unseen.

—Akbar

August 1, Year One Shortly before noon my mother-in-law, Helen, arrives at the airport in Denver, Colorado from her home in California. Her daughter Terry and I are here to meet her as she strides down the enclosed tube connecting the plane to the terminal. She is all smiles and so are we. We find her luggage, make our way out to the car, and begin our journey. For twenty minutes the conversation is so relaxed, so normal, that I begin to doubt our plan, to question what we have set in motion. And why.

"I want to take you kids out to dinner tonight," Mom offers as we rumble down the rough ribbon of asphalt.

My gut tightens a notch. With these few, utterly prosaic words, normalcy evaporates. From the back, Terry answers, her tone level, matter-of-fact.

"We can't, Mom. You'll be at the hospital."

"At the hospital?"

"Yeah, you remember. That's why we asked you to come out here."

"What?" Mom's voice rings with incredulity.

"That's why we asked you to come out here."

"Why?"

"To find out what's wrong. Why you're forgetting so much."

"Forgetting what?"

Yikes! A tough one. *"Forgetting what?" "You know." "Know what?"* *"Well, about those things." "What things?" "Those ones you don't remember."* My grip tightens on the steering wheel. I focus even harder on the road ahead and leave the answering to Terry.

"Well, you were forgetting pots on the stove. Burning things. And you were getting lost while you were driving. Remember?"

"Hmmph," Mom snorts, crossing verbal arms over her chest. "If you can remember things as good as I do when you're my age, you'll be lucky."

Two miles later, Mom points out the window toward the west. "I remember that," she says, indicating an outlet mall that did not exist when she last visited us.

We arrive at the sleek new hospital, get the tour, then head for lunch. The three of us work our way through the selections in the cafeteria, filling our trays with familiar, soothing foods. Mom half turns, facing me between the mashed potatoes and the green beans.

"Wayne, I need for you to tell me something. Do you have the keys to my suitcase?" I assure her that I do. We head for the desserts. Terry and I help Mom with the choices.

The dining area is filled with natural light but otherwise is nearly empty. We select a table near one of the many large windows. An antiseptic, weed-free expanse of lawn and a far off backdrop of mountain ranges look in on us.

"Wayne, now, you have the keys to my suitcase, don't you?" Mom asks.

"Yep, I've got 'em," I tell her, smiling and patting my front pants pocket as I come round to help her with her chair.

The Admissions Coordinator joins us. Soon we are all seated, starting on our meal, making small talk. Trying to put Mom, and ourselves, at ease.

"I just have one question," Mom announces with some urgency, interrupting an exchange of weather commentaries. "Wayne, do you know where my keys are?"

"Absolutely. I've got them right here." I fish the keys from my pocket and display them briefly. "Don't worry. I'm taking good care of them," I say, then tuck them away again, as though they belong here in her son-in-law's pocket. Mom seems satisfied. She goes back to eating, eyes down, responding only when directly addressed.

But, stabbing with her spoon at a cube of preternaturally green gelatin a few minutes later, it is obvious from the look on her face that an important question has suddenly come to mind: "I just want to know one thing, Wayne. Where are my keys?"

After lunch, Mom claws her way through the mental status exam, suffers the plunder of her purse, endures our explanations and reassurances. In the end, we leave and she remains, with nothing to cling to but her gutted handbag and our promise that we will visit tomorrow. Her plaintive wail—"Terry!"—thuds against our backs as we flee.

Evening. We call Mom at the hospital, hoping she has settled in a little, hoping she is doing well. She speaks in a furtive whisper, her voice leaking urgency and despair.

"I can't get better here," she says.

— 2 —

. . . our approach, our 'evaluations,' are ridiculously inadequate. They only show us deficits, they do not show us powers; they only show us puzzles and schemata, when we need to see music, narrative, play, a being conducting itself spontaneously in its own natural way.
—Oliver Sacks, M.D.

"It's deja vu all over again."
—Yogi Berra

August 2, Year One The Geriatric Ward representative at the hospital tells us—informally, and prior to the completion of the battery of physical, psychological, and cognitive tests Mom is undergoing—that it looks like she has dementia, depression, and delirium.

August 6 Wayne and I take Mom out of the hospital on a day pass and have dinner at The Salad Bowl. "I've been here before," Mom declares, although she has not.

She wants to go home.

August 9 Staff tell us today that my mother "will go downhill." They enumerate a long list of horrible things that will happen and say that now, at this moment, she needs 24-hour care. They offer no hope, no way out.

How can this be? Ten days ago Mom was living entirely on her own in her mobile home in California. She moved there when she was 61 years old, and has lived there for sixteen years. And for five years before that she lived alone in St. Louis, ever since my dad's— her husband, Russ's—cerebral hemorrhage. Despite the trauma of his sudden and unexpected death she did what needed doing. She made arrangements for her financial future. Within a year she sold the house she'd lived in for thirty years. She found a small rental in the neighborhood. Two years later she went through a double mastectomy and survived both the cancer and the chemo. When she was ready, she moved again, to be near my sister, Sharon, and her family. Yes, she made the move with Sharon's encouragement and with Sharon's husband, Denny, to pack the trailer and drive—but it was *she* who pulled up stakes and relocated two thousand miles across the country to San Diego County.

My mother is a person who knows her own mind. She does what she wants. She goes where she wants, when she wants. For twenty-one years she has lived life on her own terms.

And now she can't be left alone for ten minutes? What's she going to do? Burn the place down? Get lost on the way to the bathroom?

Okay, some things about her are different. She used to be an extrovert. Loved people of all ages. Talked to everyone, everywhere. When Wayne and I would meet her at the airport after a flight to visit us she always had stories to tell about her seatmates. She knew their life stories, and they, probably, hers. She was the one in the neighborhood who helped those who needed a visit, a pot of homemade soup, a driver to get to the doctor or grocery store, a companion. But somewhere along the line that began to change. Six, maybe seven years ago, she started pulling away from her neighbors at the mobile home park.

When I thought about it at all in those days, I attributed this withdrawal to her mastectomies. One day, three years after my dad's death, she found a lump in her breast. She went in for a biopsy, ended up with a mastectomy, and then a second one two days later. I never heard her complain, but on some level, I think, the loss of her breasts shook her confidence. She had a collection of prostheses, her "boobs" as she laughingly called them but, to my knowledge, she never developed or even considered an intimate relationship after her surgeries.

Slowly, my mother's social circle grew smaller. More and more she relied on Sharon, the grandkids and eventually great-grandkids, and Wayne and me, to be the people in her life.

There were other oddities, too. I remember visiting her about five years ago and noticing the calendar on her desk. The little square for every date was filled with neat but cramped writing. Not just "Dr.'s appt." or "Leona's birthday" but an accounting of the details of each day: who called, what she purchased at the store, not only whose birthday but their year of birth, their computed age, and where they live. Doubtless, this was an early storm warning, but I did not see it for what it was. My eyes saw only my neat and thorough—and perhaps a bit compulsive—mother, keeping her life in order.

One day three years ago Sharon called, upset about Mom. She was getting at least four phone calls a day from her. "But what's worse," she said, "is that she doesn't seem to know that she's already called." At Sharon's urging, Wayne and I invited Mom to visit us. She was a little eccentric, but we thought she did pretty well. We didn't see, or maybe didn't recognize, the worrisome behaviors that Sharon had described. I just figured that her sitting in front of the TV so much and not participating very actively in conversation was due to her getting old. She was in good spirits. I was satisfied that everything was all right with her.

Two years later, during an eight month period that Wayne and I lived in San Diego County, I saw things a little differently. I noticed that Mom couldn't bear to watch TV dramas anymore. She only liked the silliest, broadest comedies. She'd also apparently forgotten how to prepare her famed turkey chili. And now she called *us* four times a day, and was frequently confused about when we were coming to her home for dinner. I began to share my observations with a gerontologist friend, who helped me realize that maybe Mom wasn't just "getting old."

The next and final time we were in the area, this past May, I went to the doctor with her. Mom had always been a confident driver but now she seemed to have moved significantly along the continuum toward aggressive. She drove fast. She braked hard. I wished I were driving.

During the exam her doctor asked me to leave the room. When I returned, Mom confided to me somewhat uneasily that she hadn't been able to tell him the name of the president, "even though I voted for him." In the hallway later, the doctor told me my mother was "having memory problems" and that we should move her closer to us. I asked about a medication she was taking at the time, Halcion, whether it might be the cause of the problem or some part of it. He wondered where she got that, and told me to take it out of her house that very day. A weight descended on me. I was suddenly being put in charge of something not my own, and that was a responsibility for which I had no desire. My mother was no longer in complete control of her life.

I think she knew that she couldn't be, although she had no intention of carrying the idea to an extreme—like giving up her Halcion. She was furious that we were even discussing the subject with her, and it was embarrassing and heartbreaking to have to search out the drug, Wayne or I distracting her while the other plundered her privacy. And it was odd and angering to discover from the labels that the medication had been prescribed by the very doctor who had questioned its presence in her house. Because Mom had purchased them in blister-packs Wayne was able to exchange all of the unopened ones at the pharmacy for a refund. When he returned without the medication to face Mom's anger he led off with the handful of cash. Mom was very pleased to get the money and, to our surprise and relief, never mentioned the Halcion at all.

Wayne and I were hoping that it was medications that were causing her mental fog, and that she would soon improve now that one had been eliminated and her doctor had reduced another, Valium, to a maximum of one tablet each evening before bed.

Soon after, Wayne and I left for home in Colorado. A month ago, in July, Sharon called to say that Mom had taken a rather sudden turn for the worse. We knew of a hospital here in Colorado we thought might be able to help.

Our hope when we invited Mom here for a diagnostic work-up was that she would recover her health, go back home, and live her life.

It is still our hope.

August 11   At the Planning Conference today my mother is told that her diagnosis is "Probable Alzheimer's-type Dementia." Irreversible. No driving. No drinking. No living alone.

"My father lived to be ninety-five and didn't have this," she says, squeezing my hand as she peers across the table at these people who are directing her life. "Where would I live?" she asks of no one in particular. "Would I sell my mobile home?"

After the meeting Wayne and I decide to find a place for the three of us to live together. The problem is that two years ago we committed ourselves to working full-time to start our new writing/publishing business. To cut expenses we sold many of our belongings and household furnishings and have lived since in a dozen places, including our cabin in the mountains, the homes of friends, a travel trailer in my sister's yard, a nature preserve in California, and a high rise apartment building in Colorado.

We actually consider moving the three of us up to our cabin, but as it is located at 8,000 feet elevation, has only one room, inadequate heat, a limited amount of solar-generated electricity, and no bathroom or running water, we quickly abandon the idea and enter upon a panic search for rental housing in town.

August 14   Mid-August: the absolute worst time to find a place to rent. But somehow, in three short days we've done just that—found a two-bedroom unfurnished house on a quiet street, not too far from the business district, stores, and doctors. The price with utilities is $800+, way beyond any personal budget we have or can imagine. But it is available, and the owner is willing to let us have it on a month-to-month basis, a real plus and virtually unheard of here, where 12-month leases are the norm. We have no idea how things will turn out—whether Mom will recover and return home, whether her health will worsen in short order and she will require nursing or hospital care, whether she might die suddenly or live many years at home with need of assistance.

August 15   At the attorney's office Mom is calm and patient and cooperative. We're here to receive Power-of-Attorney from her. We need it so that we can speak for her legally in all matters. It's what we have to do. All the books and all the experts say so. Still, it's our idea, not hers. We don't know if she really understands what is taking place, but we know she understands that something important is happening. "Your dad would be sad if he knew what we were doing," she says. "He'd want to be here."

August 16   Wayne and I bring Mom to look at the house we're thinking of renting. She says she likes it. "This is a lot of trouble for you," she says. "I'd like to help out."

In fact, it is her funds which will pay the bills here. We want to tell her, to reassure her that she *is* helping out, but we don't know a way to do it that she can understand, that won't frighten and upset her. So we sign the contract in her name, pay the deposit and first month's rent from her checkbook, and prepare to care for her in a house that she believes is ours.

August 21   We drag a few things down from the cabin: a double bed for Mom, a small dining table, two molded-plastic chairs, an ancient washing machine that has been threatening to fall apart for a decade, and some basic cooking utensils. Friends—and even our new neighbors and our landlord—have loaned or given us a medley of needed household items and furnishings.

A house-filling, and a house-warming, too.

August 23   Mom sits in the middle of the living room on one of the plastic chairs. Terry rubs her shoulders and upper back, the chair swaying slightly under the rhythmic pressure.

"You're awfully cute," Mom tells her daughter's reflection in the vacant TV screen.

"I was thinking the same thing about you," Terry says.

August 25   My mother talks about going back to her mobile home. Often. She has totally forgotten that she was told she has Alzheimer's, that two weeks ago she herself talked about selling her mobile home. Now she expects to find it around every corner. She searches for it on foot. She begs us to drive her there, offers to pay us. Wayne and I take turns explaining to her that it's very far away—"more than a thousand miles" we tell her honestly—that it would take two or three long days of driving to get there.

She doesn't believe us.

August 26   This evening, a night out with Mom to celebrate our new living arrangement. Wayne and I have chosen a small café which, even though located at a bit of a distance, has a distinct attraction for us: Mom and I ate lunch there during her visit three years ago. It seems that nearly every place she has been these few weeks since her arrival in Colorado she has proclaimed, "I've been here before," despite the fact that in almost every instance she has not. Tonight she'll be right.

"I've never been here before," Mom announces happily as the three of us approach the door.

And what might be the name of this restaurant she claims never to have seen before? *Deja Vu.*

All over again.

August 28   Today is Mom's 78th birthday. I get up with her at 5 a.m. She loves it and lauds me with her new version of a compliment: "For a younger daughter you are really terrific," she exclaims. "I can't get over it."

During a phone call later, Sharon tells Mom that she is welcome to stay for a while in the camper trailer parked in their back yard if she'd like.

After the call I find that Mom has misinterpreted my sister's offer. "Sharon doesn't want me in her house now that I'm ill," she tells me. "She's afraid I'm contagious. Afraid I'll hurt the kids."

August 31   Although my mother-in-law's communications are often muddled, confusing, and sometimes unintelligible to us despite our best efforts, this is not always the case. For the most part, in fact, we all understand one another quite well and with little or no difficulty. At times, her statements are even exquisitely concise and expressive. By turns humorous, poignant, poetic; lush with metaphor and powerful imagery.

As we prepare to run some errands Mom searches her purse, finally extracting from it a piece of clear vinyl. With curious anticipation she unfolds it. It is a raincap, but a series of splits in the aged plastic render it useless now.

Mom studies the article a moment, her long fingers nimbly reading the damage. "This is what happens when you don't use things," she says, methodically refolding the hat. "This is what is going to happen to me."

September 10   Mom gets up this morning at 6 a.m., cold. I coax her back to bed and tuck her in.

"I was lying awake," she confides, "wondering if my brother Steve is alive." I reassure her that he is and hug her. "My little mother," she says. "You're my mother. I'm not your mother. I used to be your mother, but . . . other things took precedence."

September 11   Over a simple meal of soup and sandwiches Mom shares something unfathomable about the workings of her brain. Gazing out the window to the street and indicating our car parked at the curb she announces, "I think that when I bite this potato chip that car is going to move."

September 14 "How long does it take for the plane to get me to Sharon's?" my mother asks as we eat lunch and discuss her upcoming weekend trip to California for granddaughter Mimi's wedding.

"About 2½ hours," I say.

"I don't like to eat anything when I fly."

"Good, because they aren't feeding you anything."

"That's good, because it makes me sick."

"Well, you won't have to worry about that this time."

"I had food on the way out here."

"You know, you don't have to eat it when they offer you food. You can just say 'No, thanks' and they'll pass you by."

"Why would I do that?"

"If you don't want to eat on the plane."

"Honey, I'd get hungry!"

"Well, then you could eat."

"Good." Mom takes a bite of sandwich, then surveys Wayne and me with a serious gaze. "I don't know how I'm going to be able to thank you kids for all you've done for me," she says.

Wayne and I are speechless. What have we done to deserve this sudden accolade?

"And all you've undone," Mom adds. The two of us burst out laughing. Mom joins in. "I had to make that funny, didn't I?"

September 16 On the Interstate, heading to the airport:

Mom: So, in other words, she'll meet us at the airport.

Wayne: Yes. Sharon will meet you at the San Diego Airport.

M: What?

W: Sharon will meet you at the airport. In San Diego.

M: She's not going to be here to pick me up?

W: No, she's going to meet you in *San Diego*, when you get off the plane.

M: Oh, shit. I don't want to go to San Diego. I want to go to Sharon's.

W: I know. And you *are* going to Sharon's. But first you have to get to California. Then Sharon will pick you up at the airport and take you to her house.

M: I thought you said she was going to meet us here.

W: She can't. We're too far away. See, we're in Colorado. Sharon lives in California. It would take her three days to drive here.

M: (perplexed) What?

W: That's why you're taking a plane. It will get you to California in just a couple of hours.

M: I don't understand how a plane can land at Sharon's.

W: It won't. It will land in San Diego. Sharon will drive down from her house to the airport and pick you up. Then she'll take you to her house.

M: Sharon won't be here at the airport?

W: No.

M: You said she was going to meet us.

W: She'll meet you in San Diego. See, first I take you to this airport in Colorado. Then the plane goes up in the air and flies to California and lands in San Diego. Sharon will be there. Just like *I'm* taking you *to* this airport, *she'll* meet you *at* the San Diego airport and take you to her house. You'll stay in David's room.

M: How does the plane know how to get to my mobile home in California?

W: Not to your mobile home. To California.

M: How does the plane know how to get to California?

W: There's a pilot. He knows how to get there.

M: How does he know? I don't know how to get there.

W: That's his job. He does it all the time.

M: Honey, he does not. You can't land a plane at my mobile home park.

W: He won't land at your park. He'll land in San Diego. Sharon will pick you up.

M: Do you know where you're going?

W: Yep.

M: That's good. Because I don't know where in the hell I am.

W: That's okay. Stick with me. I'll get you there.

M: And Sharon will pick me up in San Diego.

W: Exactly.

M: She knows where the airport is?

W: She sure does. She'll be waiting for you when you get off the plane.

M: In other words, she's not going to meet us.

W: Not here. She'll meet you when you get off the plane.

M: I'm going to *fly?*

September 19   On the way home from the airport after her return from California Mom is in a particularly good mood. "Wayne," she says, "you know how you always tell me it's 3,000 miles to my mobile home?"

"One thousand miles. Mmmhmm."

"Denny didn't think so. He found it right away."

September 21   Deterioration of language skills and abstract thinking ability are well known symptoms of dementia. Even so, we take oral communication—especially simple, everyday interactions—so for granted that problems in this area provide unending surprise and puzzlement. They can be dangerous, they can be funny, and they can be extremely frustrating.

For some years prior to our current understanding of the scope and cause of the cognitive problems that Terry's mother is having, I found her becoming ever more obtuse and offensive in her verbal interactions. It became common for her to respond to almost any introductory sentence in a conversation with an emphatic, irritated (and irritating) *"What?"* By her response one might think that asking her if she wanted anything from the store was akin to asking if she wanted anything from the moon. Or that telling her that Sharon was on the phone—*"Who?"*—was for a moment like introducing her to a daughter she somehow didn't even know she had.

Early on, my thought was that she was becoming hard of hearing. But this theory seemed not to hold up to other observations in which her hearing appeared average to acute. More and more I came to assume that her "What?" was an intentional, lazy manipulation of those around her, although what purpose this served I could never understand.

There were other odd behaviors that crept in over the years: a compulsion to note and comment on the right- or left-handedness of those around her; a tendency to interrupt and distort conversations by turning the focus to herself; a tiring repetition of quips and jingles—"Have you driven a Ford lately? I have *never* driven a Ford!"; an endless attention to tedious details of her immediate environment while losing the thread of the conversation; the placement of periods at the ends of lines of address on envelopes.

Although in hindsight such behaviors seem like connected and glaringly obvious symptoms, at the time they seemed like nothing so much as an accumulation of old-age eccentricities and bad manners. For the most part, I was outwardly patient and forgiving. But privately, and to Terry, I wondered why her mother—so unlike the woman I had known for the previous quarter of a century—insisted on being so testy, self-centered, and mean-spirited.

When we made arrangements a month ago to live under the same roof, the frequency with which I experienced these behaviors intensified dramatically, along with my feelings of resentment. It is unflattering testimony to my own self-centeredness that her diagnosis did little to soften my judgments.

In recent days I have made a conscious effort to view her behavior differently. I do not dismiss entirely the notion that at least some portion of the communication problems we have is under her control, but I recognize, and struggle to accept, that much of it is not. It may well be also that the difficulties she experiences are so angering and frustrating to her, that she is so tired of correcting herself, so ashamed of misunderstanding and being misunderstood, that she *does* occasionally succumb to the temptation to make life a little difficult for those, like myself, who have at times been less than generous with her. Occasionally she tells me as much: "I'm just giving you a hard time." But even that may be a cover—defining her behavior as intentional, a joke, rather than having it recognized as yet one more mistake.

To the extent that I succeed in taking on this more compassionate perspective, rather than taking things personally, I find it is easier to be patient and tolerant. An unexpected discovery: patience and tolerance are not only easier on Mom, they are easier on me! Assuming good intentions rather than ill leaves me with more time and energy. I am much more alert now to catching the confusions as they come, anticipating them even, interpolating and editing for her as she speaks. I am less likely to correct her—because I see her less as "wrong"—and when I do, it is more likely to be with a gentle rephrasing, demonstrating (and checking) that I understand her meaning.

Recently I taped some colorful leaves to the wall in the living room, "They're all crisp and dry and fall-like," Terry said. "Well, of course!" Mom replied. "They're right under the heat!"

A forced-air heat register was nearby below the leaves. The leaves were not right under the heat, they were right *over* the heat. I have heard her make numerous other errors of a similar pattern—using the opposite of the word intended; getting the right words but putting them in the wrong order; transposing subject and object.

Terry and I both caught her error in this instance and responded as though she had not misstated herself. In this case it was not an important mistake. But it gives me pause. Are these merely verbal missteps, or are they part of some broader range of perceptual and processing errors? What if she is driving down the road in her 1973 Dart Swinger, as she was doing less than two months ago and as she longs to still? Might she mistake left for right, stop for go, accelerator for brake?

It is my habit to take another's words at face value. It is difficult, indeed impossible, always to catch another's mistakes, to read between misspoken and unspoken lines, to ferret out intended meaning.

And it is tiring. Might it not one day prove altogether exhausting?

September 24 Mom tells Wayne and me today, "It's a darn shame I can't live in my mobile home where I so desperately want to be."

September 26 Mom has watched *Guiding Light* for as long as I can remember. And she has carried her habit into her new home with us, where it has provided a welcome link to all those yesterdays.

Today, in the midst of the program she exclaims, "I've been watching my soap opera so long now I almost know what's going on!"

September 28 With purple dusk still tinting the windows, my mother readies herself for bed. It is just past 7:30 p.m., her usual hour now, though when she lived alone she was always a late-nighter. She always had a small array of medications by her bed then. Now, she turns to me for such things.

Tonight she asks me for a Tylenol. "So that I can go to sleep," she says. Wayne and I have substituted Tylenol for Valium, which she took for many years prior to coming to us. Mom doesn't seem to mind, and sleeps better now than I've ever known her to. This night I suggest prayer, knowing that she always enjoyed praying at bedtime.

"I can't remember any," she says.

"Make them up," I encourage. "That's the best kind."

I tuck her in—another role-reversal ritual, one that we both enjoy—kiss her forehead, tell her that I love her.

"I love *you*," she says. "More than you know." She says it with a beautiful, sparkling smile. "You're a good kid," she adds suddenly.

Like a mom.

Much madness is divinest sense
To a discerning eye.

—Emily Dickinson,
J. 435

"He's singing in shorthand."

—Helen

October 4, Year One Wayne and I are scheduled for a half-day school visit today. Presenting our writing program at schools is a major part of our work and livelihood, and this first school visit of the year is here in town. Mom is nervous about the prospect of being alone all afternoon. She wants the phone numbers of our neighbor Ella, Sharon, and the school.

October 11 After listening to a TV news story about adoption Mom asks, "Did you adopt me?" Before Wayne or I can speak she supplies her own answer: "Well, you adopted me for a while."

October 20 My mother has always loved music. She sang professionally in her early twenties before she married. When I was young, she would sing all the songs from her night club performances as she worked around the house. The family's favorite time to listen to her sing was while riding in the car. For that very reason, my father even refused to have a radio installed.

Her favorite singers have always been Perry Como and Bing Crosby. In recent years her affection for Perry Como has taken on an almost obsessive quality. Her cassette tape player has become her greatest source of entertainment.

Her current favorite recording by Mr. Como, "Just Out Of Reach," was left behind in California. Wayne has managed a rustic version on his guitar, much to Mom's delight, but we ordered a new record a few weeks ago just the same, which arrived in today's mail. Only now does it occur to us that we have no turntable on which to play the 45rpm disk. Mom doesn't seem to mind. In fact, she is ecstatic. When I ask her at lunch, "What do you want on your sandwich?" she holds the record in her outstretched hands, as though the better to take it all in, and says, "I don't need anything, now that I have my record. This is the best day of the year!"

Did I say *almost* obsessive?

October 31 Mom is alone in her room. "I'm sorry you're dead," I hear her say. "I hope you have a good time. I told you I'm a little nuts."

"I have everything I want at my mobile home," she tells me later, "except your father."

A photo of my father sits by her bed. Was it to him she was speaking earlier?

November 6 The three of us watch a news story about Ronald Reagan's Alzheimer's diagnosis. "I feel sorry for him," Mom says, "because he has that disease."

November 20 Six a.m. Mom emerges from her room singing, "Oh what a beautiful morning!" as though she is making an entrance on stage.

In mid-morning Mom and I meet Wayne and a young neighbor boy at the library. Mom's mood has changed. "I'd rather be at home standing on my head than be here!" she announces in a voice loud enough for many of the patrons and staff to hear. I seethe as I drive Mom home. When we arrive, I leave her there and go to a friend's house to give myself a chance to cool off.

An hour later I return. By coincidence, Wayne arrives at the same time after having taken our neighbor home. We enter the house to find Mom in the kitchen, sweeping industriously. Three of the four electric burners on the range top are glowing full red. The room is sprayed with shards of glass and a gooey, unidentified substance.

"I was just trying to heat up the pie," Mom explains, her voice trembling with guilt and fear, her broom still flailing at the glass.

It takes some time to piece the story together: home alone, Mom decided to have some pie for a snack. Warm pie would be nice, so she placed the glass pie plate with its one remaining piece of cherry pie directly on the electric burner. Unsure which knob controlled which burner, she tried several, soon sending a barrage of shrapnel across the kitchen. By a stroke of luck she was not injured, but she was shaken, and remains so even now.

Angry and in need of a respite, we left her alone for one hour. This is the result.

We, too, are filled with guilt and fear.

Thanksgiving Mom tells my friend Jean that she will stay with Wayne and me until she's well enough to go back home. She has a bladder infection, she explains. An inaccurate statement, although one I have heard her share with others as well.

I wonder, is this her explanation to the world, and to herself, about the recent changes in her life?

November 29 My mother tells me that I am sometimes critical of her. This is very accurate. I have been trying to fix her, trying to set her straight about the many things she gets wrong. I think it's fear that makes me impatient and angry with her. Fear of the future. She picks up on my fear and anger, and feels insecure and stupid.

At dusk lately she has been seeing rain. Every evening she stands at the living room window, calls me or Wayne over and, in a voice filled with dismay, urges, "Look at that rain."

But it's not raining. Every time, it's not raining. She wants me to agree with her; I can hear the plea in her voice. But I'm afraid to, afraid that agreeing will somehow make her sicker. Or that it will make me sick, too.

"No," I say again this evening, "I can't see it." I ease the words out, trying to allow by my tone that my failure to see the rain is not a final word on the matter. Mom reads me just right, and meets me halfway in return.

"You're blind," she says. "But you're smart."

November 30   As I leave for the post office, my mother-in-law hands me an envelope, eagerly directing my attention to the "address" she has written on it:

I watch my favorite news man
Tom Brokaw. From Monday night through
Friday night
at Clevedon Street

"Mom," I say hesitantly, "I don't think this will get to Tom Brokaw." At first she is confused, is still caught up in the elation of having found "Tom Brokaw" in the *TV Guide* after searching for the listing all morning.

"Oh," she says, suddenly seeing my point. "That will be delivered here."

Or nowhere.

I open the envelope later. It's a Christmas card. Inside the card is a photo of our TV playing Tom Brokaw on the evening news. This is not particularly surprising to me. Mom takes many photographs of people on television, and also takes photographs of photographs. As far as Terry and I can tell, she considers her subjects to be living, breathing people who are physically in her presence. But, curiously, the photos she takes of them, once printed, she considers to be just that: photographs.

December 1 "What's the date, Wayne?" Mom asks me.
"December 1st."
A bit later, I go to the calendar that hangs on the kitchen wall and turn the page from November to December. In the square with the "1", in Mom's bold lettering, I find this notation:

TODAY.

It is a far cry from her calendar notations of a few years ago. Yet the humanity embodied in this ineffectual inscription fills it with meaning, though only for me, not for Mom. It tells me more about her condition, and the purity and tenacity of her spirit, than any room full of doctors or any shelf full of books ever will. It is a meditation. A poem, with apologies to Paul Simon, composed of five letters.

December 13 Mom is searching through the *TV Guide* for Bing Crosby's movie, *White Christmas*. "You can see people who are dead on television," she explains.

December 14 *White Christmas* is on. Mom is psychic!

December 15 *White Christmas* yesterday, *Perry Como's Irish Christmas* special today. Mom is transported. When Perry Como sings "Ave Maria" she explains to Wayne and me with reverent wonder, "He's singing in shorthand."

December 20 Mom comes with us on a half-day author-visit to another local elementary school. The teachers look out for her when she gets bored and starts wandering the halls during our presentations.
We eat in the teachers' lunchroom. Mom hoards food and loads snacks and sweets into her purse. No one complains.

December 21 We're getting Mom packed and ready to leave for Sharon's tomorrow. She will spend Christmas there and then Wayne and I will come in mid-January to live with her in her mobile home for two months while we bring our enrichment programs to schools in southern California.

December 22 Mom is up at 5 a.m., happy and expectant. "You're like my mother," she tells Terry, who packs a suitcase for her. "You're so organized."

I drive her to Denver, once again to catch a plane to San Diego. But this trip is much different than three months ago. While our conversation is not deep, it is better described by the word "normal" than any other. Mom has little trouble understanding the whole scenario this time around: we drive to Denver; she flies to San Diego; Sharon picks her up there.

As I write these words I am struck by how well Mom is doing, at least in comparison to a few months ago. Is she getting better? Or is it part of the fluctuation we have seen before: encouraging hours or days followed by hope-dashing periods of seemingly major regression?

December 30 Mom calls from Sharon's, crying. Missing Wayne, missing the snow, missing our neighbor Ella, missing me.

— 4 —

"I'm so tired of being confused all the time."

—Helen

January 11, Year One   Terry and I arrive in San Diego County. We have dinner at Sharon and Denny's house. Mom has heard from them that she and Terry and I will be staying at her mobile home, and she is eager.

January 13   In preparation for Mom's move in, Wayne and I have spent two days cleaning the trailer, stocking food, and clearing out nineteen grocery bagfuls of poisons, caustic cleaners, and general clutter (including possibly every bank statement, cancelled check, phone bill, grocery and pharmacy receipt she has ever received in California).

We also find boxes filled with memories: photos and letters she has cached throughout the trailer. Who would have thought that 550 square feet could cradle so much of a life?

January 14   Our first night together. Wayne and I need some semblance of privacy. Mom doesn't seem to. We put her good mattress on the fold-out couch in her living room; Wayne and I will sleep on the couch's thin foam mattress on her box spring in the only bedroom.

After a middle-of-the-night trip to the bathroom Mom turns right, toward the bedroom, rather than left toward the living room. She is surprised, though not alarmed, to find people in her bed.

"Mom," I call quietly, trying to orient her, to get her attention. "Mom."

Finally, she recognizes that it is me. "I can't . . . find . . . where I . . . want to go," she says.

It is as much a struggle for her to get through the sentence as to figure out where she is, and why her daughter is in her bedroom. All of this strikes her funny bone, and mine, too. We giggle like schoolgirls on a sleep over.

January 16   Yesterday morning Mom declared, "I want to go to the other place." I thought she meant the house in Colorado.

But today, standing in the kitchen of the mobile home in which she lived for sixteen years prior to coming to Colorado six months ago, she insists again that she wants to go to "the other place." Through a Twenty Questions-like process Wayne and I come to understand that she means her mobile home. This mobile home. After all her many weeks of wishing for it, here she stands and still longs for it.

"This isn't it," she says. "I know where it is, but I can't find it. I've been confused since your father died so suddenly. I don't understand it."

"I don't either," I say, and we cry together.

January 17   Mom says she's "tired of all the crap" she gets from Sharon and me. (Hey, wait a minute! What about from Wayne?) And she's obsessed about finding the other place. Again and again she insists that this is not her mobile home. She knows this for a certainty because, "Where I used to live I could find my way to church."

January 24   Mom smiles all day over new-found treasures of old photographs, cards, and letters. All the while, Perry Como sings in the background.

January 28   David, Mom's nine year old great-grandson, has come to spend the night. He bunks down on the floor in the living room, not far from Mom's bed, in his cartoon character-decorated sleeping bag.

"You don't have to sleep all alone in this big room," Mom assures him. "I'll be here. If you need anything in the night, wake me up."

January 29   Mom enjoyed David's overnight visit. But this morning she tells Terry, "Thanks for cooking for the little kid and taking care of him." Sometimes she seems to understand her situation. And, in her way, to acknowledge.

I take Mom on a drive so that she can "find her other place." I drive a long distance, through much of north San Diego County for an hour and a half, taking every turn she requests, all to no avail. Tempers grow short. We exchange epithets.

February 4   My mother ate a huge piece of chocolate cake and lots of candy at her granddaughter Mimi's baby shower an hour ago. Back at her trailer now, she is the most confused I have ever seen her in my life. She doesn't remember that Sharon and Denny are married or that Denny is Mimi's father.

"Does Mimi know?" she asks. "Am *I* her mother?"

"No, you're her grandma."

"Why didn't anyone tell me?" she rages. Even when she accepts my memory she is no less angry or pained. "This is a real slap in the puss," she says, and cries softly for herself. "I'm so tired of being confused all the time."

Soon, she finds a way out of her misery: "I'm more in love with Perry Como than ever," she says.

February 18   Ever since she came to Colorado in August Mom has missed driving. She talked about her car quite a lot at first, although that faded with time and with her growing fondness for our car, with its cassette player capable of playing Perry Como tapes.

Now that we are here at her mobile home her interest in her car is rekindled. The object of her affection, a 1973 Dodge Dart Swinger (with air conditioning!), holds great sentimental value for her as it was an anniversary gift from my dad just a few months before he died.

One of the recurrent anxieties we experience living here with Mom is that her car still sits in this driveway. For more than a month we have kept its doors locked, refused her requests for the keys— which infuriates her (and why not?)—and distracted her as best we could whenever she has made mention of it.

Today Wayne has the bright idea to disconnect the battery, which will allow us to give her the keys and still prevent the possibility of her taking off to terrorize southern California. But it isn't necessary—the battery is dead. Hardly surprising in a 20-year old vehicle that has been sitting unused for six months. Why didn't we check before?

When next she asks about the car, we gladly give her the keys. She goes out, struggles to open the unlocked driver's door, and slides behind the wheel. We peer from behind parted curtains as she cranes her neck back and forth, studying the interior, searching for the past. Twice she passes her hand tenderly across the vinyl seat back, then gets out, returns to the house, and hangs the key ring on its familiar nail. She says nothing, but we know that it is finished.

This is what we so feared. This is what we struggled to deny her.

February 22   Mom's new great-granddaughter was born today. She is very gentle with Katie, holding her on her lap, cradling her head, and talking to her like great-grandmothers have since they were invented.

February 25   Since the day of her diagnosis last summer, when the hospital doctors advised my mother-in-law against alcohol consumption, we have dutifully and successfully kept her from the clutches of demon rum. This, despite her having consumed alcohol regularly when her husband was alive, and despite her having been an avid fan of wine with dinner until the day she arrived in Colorado. It has been a surprisingly quiet revolution: she has never once asked for wine, and has instead become an enthusiastic consumer of the apple and cranberry juices which we provide.

Yesterday, however, we received a shot across our bow when Mom stopped with Sharon at a familiar store and found her way to the liquor aisle. She purchased a large bottle of wine, guarded the cargo on the return trip to her mobile home, and unloaded it out of the van here, warning Terry, Sharon, and me, "Don't touch this or I'll kill you."

While I think none of us took this threat quite literally, she was clearly not in a negotiating mood. Moreover, the set of her jaw and the steely glint in her eye as she escorted the brown-papered jug up the steps and through the sliding door were potent reminders that her mind, memory, and emotions are less stable than they used to be. Once inside, she promptly buried her treasure in a wicker basket by her bedside.

Today we find it in the back of the refrigerator. Still in its paper bag. Still unopened.

March 4 "Comb your hair. My guys can see you," Mom says as I come into the living room.

The "guys" she is referring to are two magazine covers propped against a chair back, one featuring Johnny Carson, the other with three photos of NFL players. I don't want to hear what her paper people think.

"I don't care," I say.

She digests this for a moment. "You have a husband," she says then. "I have nothing."

Instantly, understanding dawns and my irritation falls away. "So you'd rather have paper than nothing?"

"Yeah," she says, the tension melting from her face. "They smile and I smile back. It's fun."

March 6 A vase full of red and pink roses adorns the trailer. Mom's been cutting flowers lately, from wherever she finds them around the mobile home park.

"I want to be a real old lady," she tells me as though announcing a new-found vocation, "and be able to walk."

March 9 Terry and I break the news to Mom of our upcoming departure on a business trip to visit schools in western Colorado. Our worry is that she won't want to move to Sharon's and live there until our tour is completed and we can all return to our Colorado house in April. Our worry is that she will want to stay in her mobile home.

"I'll be here alone," Mom says in a tone that sounds like anticipation.

"Oh, Mom, you don't want to live here all alone," I say hurriedly. She sits on the couch/bed; her fingers fidget with the spread.

"Mom, we don't want you to stay alone here," Terry says.

An old lady, her face knotted in puzzlement, looks a long moment at her daughter. When she speaks her words are forlorn, tinged with fear: "I don't even know how to lock my door."

"Well, see, that's what we mean," I say. "Besides, there's been a break-in here at the park," I add ominously. It's the truth, but I despise myself for playing on her insecurity.

"I wouldn't want to be around here for that," Mom says.

We tell her of Sharon's invitation to stay with them while Terry and I are traveling. "Where would I sleep?" she asks. "In David's bed?"

"Yes," Terry says. "And you can watch your Perry Como video," she quickly adds.

"How can I watch it?" Mom asks.

"On Sharon and Denny's VCR."

"What's that?"

March 13 We took Mom to Sharon's last night. This morning, while doing a final cleaning at the mobile home prior to our departure, Wayne discovers once again Mom's precious bottle of wine in the refrigerator. Although three weeks have passed, it has not been opened, moved, or mentioned since the day she placed it there.

The phone rings. I answer it, and am startled to hear my mother's voice on the line. To simplify things last night we explained to her that we were leaving on our trip, implying that our departure was then and there, from Sharon's house, and now I feel caught in our "lie." A strange, powerful surge of guilt and panic shoots through me, but it is unnecessary, for two reasons.

First, last night's lie was a benevolent one. Any attempted explanation of our need for time to prepare for the trip—to clean the trailer, pack the car—would have been incomprehensible to Mom. We knew that and did not trouble her with it. Second, Mom does not feel that she has "caught" me in anything. Quite the opposite. She simply wants to talk to me and is glad to hear my voice. She almost certainly has no idea of where I am and probably has little or no memory of the details of our conversation yesterday.

Mom is living in the moment. She is at Sharon's. We aren't. She took action to find us. She succeeded. She is happy.

— 5 —

We are not alone.

—Wayne

We are not alone, and we are having fun.

—Helen

March 14, Year One On this return trip to Colorado Terry and I have several school visits scheduled, arranged during these past two months in California from my temporary "office" in Mom's mobile home. This is desperately needed work and income. Our business needs our full-time attention, but does not get it because we give most of it to Mom, who needs it, too.

When making my contacts with schools I often had to leave a message and a return telephone number—in this case, Mom's number at her mobile home. Although we were there with her most of the time, it was possible that a return call might come in on one of the days we were on site at a school locally and that Mom, alone in the trailer, might answer the phone. Consequently, I took extra time to explain to each principal or receptionist I spoke with that if I were not available at the time of a return call my mother-in-law might answer and agree to take a message. *Under no circumstances*, I explained, should they believe anything she told them, no matter how polite or dependable she might sound. This was a most difficult task for me. I feared that at best I was portraying an unflattering image of our "office help" and therefore of ourselves, and that at worst I was making my mother-in-law out to be a deranged ax-murderer.

What I found, however, surprised me. In every instance, the message-taker quickly grasped what I was struggling to convey so discreetly. Many even interrupted me. "I understand exactly what you're saying," they assured me.

It was the first dawning for Terry and me of an important realization: we are not alone.

March 31   "Mom's spacy," Sharon tells me when I call after the close of a week of school visits in St. Louis. "She's trying to feed cookies and oranges to photos of you and Wayne, and to the picture of Perry Como."

Mom gets on the phone. "I'm upset," she tells me.

"Why, Mom?"

"Because half my clothes are at Sharon's other house."

A new mutation of The Other House dilemma. "I'll take care of it," I tell her, and although my statement has no literal meaning, it carries the perfect emotional message to Mom.

"Okay," she says. I can hear her relief through the wires.

In the past my usual strategy would have been to explain the truth of things, to clear up her confusion. This almost never worked. It just made her feel stupid and wrong.

The fact is that no amount of truth-telling will help my mother understand that Sharon doesn't have another house wherein are hidden half of her clothes. Intellectual understanding is not something I can give her. What she needs is not abstract understanding, but reassurance. By simply saying, "I'll take care of it," I have, at least for the moment. Which is all there is.

April 13   Mom returned to Colorado today. She was very animated through the evening, talking to Terry and me nonstop, exploring and reacquainting herself with her room and the house in general.

And she's keeping us awake tonight, too, talking and laughing with her friends—the photos on her bedroom walls.

April 14 My mother-in-law can be startlingly abrasive at times, and excruciatingly polite at others. "Shut up," she has demanded on more than one occasion, "Tom Brokaw is on." Another time she barked at me, "Stop talking. Our president is speaking." But, in the car today she coaxed ever so gently, "Wayne, if you would turn the radio just a little louder you could hear Perry Como singing very distinctly."

Her attachment to and personification of inanimate images, which we now realize began while she was still living on her own, has intensified steadily over the past eight months. Objects of her affection include an Ozzie Smith refrigerator magnet; *TV Guide* covers; a toothpaste ad featuring a cherubic young girl's smiling, toothy face; family photographs; a framed picture of her husband. And Perry Como.

Last winter we ordered a videotape of the *Perry Como's Irish Christmas* special which she enjoyed so much when it was broadcast on TV. She still watches the video on a regular basis, but the video *box*, which features a smiling, relaxed Perry, has become her constant companion. She treats it like a him, not an it, talking to him, bringing him with her on walks and outings in the car.

She calls him by a variety of names: my guy, the kid, Perry, Perry Como's brother. Today he's "the priest" and he joins us for dinner. Mom is excited and tries to feed the box yams and apple juice. Finally she gives up. "He just smiles," she says contentedly.

Later, she summarizes her world in a post card to a friend: "We are not alone, and we are having fun."

April 19 Every day Mom goes for multiple walks around the neighborhood, often with her guy, Perry Como. The exercise, fresh air, and mental stimulation are good for her; the minutes alone are salvation for us. Lately she's been bringing back grape hyacinth and sprigs from blossoming plum trees. We tell ourselves the neighbors don't mind.

April 21   Mom enjoyed the library today. I enjoyed it less after she found an ad which she liked in a magazine, promptly and loudly ripped it out, folded it, and placed it in her purse.

I think I could handle living with and caring for my mother a lot better if I weren't attached to helping her. One source of my attachment is duty: I want to help her because I "owe" it to her; I owe it to her because she *is* my mother. Another source of my attachment is that I want something back: her love, attention, and regard.

Today I make this prayer and promise: Helen, I release you completely. Please forgive me, as I forgive myself, for trying to make you be a certain way. I forgive you for doing the same with me.

Just love her.

April 22   Remarking on her framed photograph of my dad (a 3/4 pose), Mom complains, "Your father won't look at me."

April 26   Snow fell last night. This morning, Mom and I have a snowball fight and then, together, we ambush Wayne. Mom says it's the most fun she's had in a long time. I remind her of the figure-eights that she's always told me she did as a kid, skating on the pond near her home.

"If I had done a figure-nine," she explains now with unassailable logic, "I would have gone off the lake."

April 27   She puts a newspaper article in an envelope, seals it, and places it under the *Irish Christmas* video with a note which says, "Read when you have the time." Later, she points out that Perry hasn't read it, which she knows because the envelope hasn't been opened.

April 28   "Sometimes when I talk to your dad's picture," Mom says, "it's almost as if he can hear me." Later, referring to the Perry Como box, she clearly views the world differently. "I wonder if we could find a doctor for him," she says. "To find out why he doesn't talk."

May 3 Tired of waiting at a regularly scheduled appointment with her (real) doctor, Mom suddenly announces to everyone in the clinic waiting room, "If they think I'm here for my health, they're nuts."

May 15 Mom is excited about our imminent trip to New Mexico, and has been since Terry and I first broached the subject with her several months ago. She's eager to go to the places she saw on her honeymoon. And to visit her older brother, Joe, his wife, Nettie, and their son and daughter-in-law.

Early on, she mistook our mention of the possibility of a trip as a cue to start packing. Since then, feeling assured that she is genuinely interested, we have made plans without Mom's further input or knowledge. When she does bring it up we handle it with the type of reassuring but attention-diverting response that has more and more become second-nature to us:

"Oh, yeah, that'll be fun. But that's not for a while yet. Say, Mom, I'm going to the bank. Want to come along?"

"Sure. Soon as I find my guy."

May 18 We stop for lunch at The Garden Of The Gods in southern Colorado. My mother doesn't show any sign of remembering being here on her honeymoon—fifty-six years ago this week—although she revels in the beauty of the place.

We cross into New Mexico, the late afternoon sunlight glancing off the hood like a flat stone off still water. "What do you have against my brother?" Mom suddenly demands. Judging by her tone, she is furious, although I did not know that a moment ago, and have no idea why.

"What do you mean?" I say. "I have nothing against your brother."

"Then why aren't we staying there?"

"At Joe's?"

"Yes, at Joe's," she snaps.

I explain to Mom—even as I struggle to quell the anger that has risen now in me as well—that we have not been invited to stay at

Joe and Nettie's, but at the home of their son. I calmly remind her that her brother and Nettie live in a very small apartment. "They don't have any extra room," I explain. This is not new information. Mom's brother and his wife have rented their small apartment continuously since the 1950's. Mom has obviously forgotten this detail, even though on several trips to New Mexico prior to her illness she stayed not at her brother's but at her nephew's.

And now I'm being accused of having something against her brother.

* * * * *

As I silently witness this exchange between Terry and her mother, I am taken back two decades to my training and work in the fields of mental health and education. In those days, in staffings or progress notes, the words "unprovoked" and "unprecipitated" were commonly used to describe behaviors of patients or clients which were judged by the observer to be negative or undesirable. The terms were not merely descriptive; they carried heavy pejorative connotations and their use tended to impugn and marginalize the person described. The individual making such a judgment—often in a position of higher status or holding power of some kind over the person being described—had decided, and may truly have believed, that there was no worthy or sufficient cause for the behavior in question, or, in some cases, that there was no cause for it whatsoever. This exchange between Terry and her mom reminds me of the arbitrary arrogance of those stances which, twenty years ago, I took for granted to be legitimate and "correct."

What I can say today is that sometimes I do not like the way my mother-in-law behaves. Sometimes I do not understand *why* she behaves in a certain way. In the moments following her outburst, her anger seemed to me entirely without cause. It seemed to me unprecipitated. Without provocation.

But in those moments I was wrong. From Mom's perspective it's obvious: by mentioning her nephew, Terry and I abruptly and unilaterally changed the focus and purpose of our trip, which, in her mind, is to visit Joe and Nettie. Neither her question nor the emotion behind it were illogical or unprecipitated. They were provoked.

May 20   On Saturday morning we drive to Santa Fe's Old Town Plaza. Wayne and I make a strategic decision to distract Mom into leaving her picture of Perry Como in the car, hoping that familiar cues—the ancient adobe buildings, the handcrafted silver and turquoise jewelry neatly laid out on American Indian blankets, the whole aura of the place—will kindle happy memories of her visits here through the past half century.

They do not. Just as Mom did not remember Garden Of The Gods, neither does she remember the Plaza. What she remembers is Perry Como, and she is angry at Wayne for leaving him behind in the car. Tension mounts throughout the morning, as though our every labored step through the streets of this historic city winds some unseen spring. We are distraught and distracted. While crossing a street we are nearly run over by a car.

* * * * *

Everything Terry and I try is wrong, nothing works. I'm mad at Mom, she's mad at me. It's hot.

We spot an arts and crafts fair across the street. Mom is oblivious, but Terry and I are drawn to it like desert wanderers to water. We step off the curb, my attention fixed on the oasis of trees, green grass, and smiling crowds.

Suddenly a blur of metal slashes across our path not three feet in front of us. A horn drones and insults are hurled at us from the passenger and rear windows of a war-worn sedan. I respond with curses and an obscene gesture, challenging the lot of them. Tail lights flash as the driver taps the brake. Fine with me. An opportunity to slug somebody, to *be* slugged, even—one sounds as good as the other right now—doesn't seem like something to pass up.

Uniformed police are only yards away, directing traffic. They remain cool-headed, defuse the situation, and the car slips back into traffic.

Mom finds nothing entertaining at the fair and takes only temporary comfort in the cool, sweet distraction of a nearby ice cream shop. Finally, having exhausted the attractions of Santa Fe, we retreat from the city square. Soon we are trudging up the steps to St. Francis Cathedral, not only for rest and a respite from the heat, but in some desperate, agnostic way, to pray—for deliverance, for wisdom, for whatever we can get. Mom prays that I will go get Perry; her prayers are answered.

In the afternoon we escape the disappointments of Mom's forgotten honeymoon city and hunker down in the flickering gloom of a Saturday matinee. Mom explains the story to Perry as it goes along. After the film, in the parking lot and the glare of day, she is distracted and anxious and refuses to get into the car "until he joins us." Terry points out to her that she is holding the video box photo in her hand, but to no avail. It's a stand off for fifteen minutes, until patience finally wins the day and Mom slips onto the seat.

Or perhaps he joined us.

May 22   The trip has been a mini-disaster of unfulfilled expectations. All Wayne's and mine.

Mom began insisting on going home the evening we arrived and has been ready to leave every day since. This morning, having spent an excruciating four days on this long-anticipated pleasure trip, Wayne and I revamp our plans: we are leaving—now.

Mom takes this occasion to announce, "Dad is dead. This is my wedding day. I'm going to marry *him*." She points with blushing-bride pride to her ever-present picture of Perry Como. We are so discouraged, disappointed, and exhausted that this results in yet another argument, one laced generously with expletives. Mom walks out the front door with her new groom. We let her walk. We *want* her to walk. Go ahead, Mom. Walk. Walk down the aisle. Get married. Be happy. Just keep walking.

Wayne and I fume in our hosts' house for fifteen minutes. We revel in self-pity while we pack the car, congratulating each other on our righteousness. But when Mom doesn't return, the gold of our anger turns to the dross of fear. Now we walk; walk and jog the unfamiliar streets until we find her, strolling, in a pleasant mood, only a few blocks away, a sprig of lilacs in her hand.

On the return trip to Colorado we take a different route for the initial portion, meandering along state highways, rolling through picturesque foothills and forested areas, and meeting one last time with my aunt and uncle at a small natural spring where they travel regularly to fill a score of bottles with drinking water. We share a light meal together, take a few photos. Whatever may have fallen short on this trip, Mom has thoroughly enjoyed her visits with her brother and sister-in-law, who have been relaxed and loving and entirely nonplused by her condition and behavior. In fact, Mom has been more "normal" and happy in their company than with anyone else these several days. Including Wayne and me.

May 23 Wayne and I are still weary from the trip. This morning Mom wants to know, "When are we going to Santa Fe?"

Are we not always living the life
that we imagine we are?

—Henry David Thoreau

May 24, Year One   My mother called me a bitch today. Because I don't see her "guy."

May 25   She insists again this evening on bringing her guy to the table, setting a place, and feeding him. But when she wants to move the whole show to her bedroom we draw a line and flatly disallow it. Although it is I who make the strongest statement, Mom turns her anger on Terry.

"You're just a bitch," she says, the words spewing from her mouth like venom. She stands, picks up her plate of food, reaches for that of her friend.

"That's enough," I say. "I've had enough of that out of you."

Mom immediately assumes a submissive tone and posture. "I've never called her that before," she says meekly.

Not since yesterday, I want to say. I remember, even if you don't. "Well, I don't want to hear it again. It's about time you learn to behave."

I am stunned at what my ears hear from my own mouth. Grieved, too, and not only at my meanness but at my lack of originality. In an instant I have become the worst kind of parent—domineering, bullying, and condescending. Tense seconds pass; the crisis eases. Mom again picks up a plate. We ignore her and she takes it to her room.

Terry is furious. She gives no quarter for dementia and tells me over and over that she will not take her mother's abusiveness any more. She goes to bed early. I barricade myself at the TV. There are no "Good night"s this night.

* * * * *

Wayne is still in the living room when Mom knocks at my bedroom door. I open and there she is, eager and alert.

"I want to talk to you," she says in an urgent whisper.

"Okay," I say, outwardly calm but inwardly worried about what's coming next, worried that the slightest spark will set me ablaze again.

"I'm all packed," she says.

We go to her room. She points to a few items pushed together in the middle of her bed. No clothes, just the important things: her purse, her guy, her comb. I put my arms around her, pull her close.

"I want to make up but I don't think you do," she says.

"I do, Mom. I'm holding you. I want to make up." We breathe and hold. Breathe and hold. "If you aren't happy here," I tell her softly, gently as I am able, "Wayne and I will help you find a place. We want you to be happy."

"Would it be all right if I stay here tonight?"

"Mo-om,"—I'm laughing, can't help it—"even if you want to go, you don't have to go right away. You don't go tonight."

"Okay," Mom says. "I'll stay tonight."

"Good. Okay then."

Unpacking shouldn't take long.

May 28 After an hour of fruitless efforts to feed the Perry Como video box at dinner, Mom is suddenly done with him. For now. "I wonder if he can take a bus home?" she says. "I can't take him."

My friend April, who works with people who have dementia, has been encouraging Wayne and me not to challenge Mom, but to recognize that behavior is always directed toward fulfilling a need.

Because Mom can't always clearly express her needs in words, our job is to discover them, however hidden, and help her meet them. This will take some thought, and work.

June 1   Terry is away for the day. "Do you want to take a walk with me, Mom?" I ask.

"Sure." But by the time we reach the curb she is very angry with me. "Well, aren't we going?" she wants to know.

"Yeah," I say, uncertain about what has happened. "We're going. Come on." I offer her my arm and lean in the direction of the alley and its beckoning lilacs.

"I want to go in this," Mom says, pointing to our 4WD International Travelall, hulking like Gargantua at the curb.

"Mom, we're going on a walk, remember? To see the flowers."

"No. I want to go in this."

"But the flowers are right here, Mom." I point to them, barely a dozen steps from where we stand. "We can't take a 6,000 pound vehicle to see flowers across the street."

She continues to insist that I drive her to where the flowers are and I continue to refuse.

"Oh the hell with it," she says and goes back in the house. Shortly after, she comes out again, ready to walk. And we do.

At supper Mom wants to know what our friends will eat. "I'm making chili for you and me," I tell her. She brings an image of Perry Como to the table and spends the entire meal tending to it, even more so than to feeding herself. When she asks a question, I respond. "I'm talking to *him*," she explains brusquely.

Later, she asks another question, which I do not hear clearly. "Are you talking to me?" I ask.

"Yes."

Her innocent answer ignites a sudden anger in me. "Well," I say, "how am I supposed to know the difference?"

June 3   **TV:** I'm Tom Brokaw. I'll see you back here again tomorrow night.

Mom: I'm Helen. . . . At least I used to be.

June 5 Tonight Mom again wants to take food to her room to
feed Perry Como.

"You can't," Terry tells her.

"The hell I can't."

"You can bring him out here," I offer, "but eating and drinking
have to be done at the table."

She stands, tosses her silverware onto her plate, apparently in
preparation for taking it to her bedroom. "Where is he?" she asks
Terry.

"I don't see him," Terry says. Her fork dangles listlessly from
one hand.

"You're a bitch," Mom snarls.

In an instant I boil over. I get up, rush round to her side of the
table and fling my arm down over her plate, preventing her from
picking it up. "Don't talk to Terry like that," I bark.

"She's my daughter. I'll talk to her any way I want."

"No! You won't! And you're not taking food back to anybody.
There's nobody there. It's cardboard, Mom. It's not real. You can't
feed paper."

"You don't know what you're talking about."

"No. That's *you*, Mom." My rage is still building, frightening me
a little, but I don't even try to control it. I'm enjoying it. "*You're* the
one who's all mixed up. And if you keep this up they're going to
take you away." She tries to tug the plate free. I clench my hand into
a fist and shake it threateningly, inches from her face. "They're going
to . . . put you someplace . . . because . . . you have no brain! You
don't know what you're doing. It's a picture, Mom. IT'S A PIC-
TURE. So knock it off!"

Suddenly drained, I turn away. Mom retreats quickly to her
room. Terry goes to ours a moment later, and I see the hurt and
disappointment, the fear on her face. Alone in the tiny, silent room,
I slump to the floor. On the table our three unfinished dinners cool
to paste.

For twenty minutes I play the scene over and over in my head, wallowing in a quicksand fantasy of catastrophe and total ruination of everything the three of us have experienced and accomplished to this moment. I have no hope for the future. I am worthless. Stupid. Beyond forgiveness.

Terry returns, her voice soft and soothing. With her encouragement I knock on Mom's door. When she answers I tell her through the cautious crack, "I'm sorry, Mom. Can you forgive me?"

"I forgive you," she says, pulls the door wider and extends her hand. We shake on it, smile, tell one another that we love each other.

I don't know whether she forgives me because she is a generous, forgiving soul, or simply because she has forgotten.

Nor do I care. My only care is that she does.

June 25   The three of us take a drive up to the cabin. The meadow is a carpet of wildflowers. Mom sings, "The hills are alive . . ." When we arrive she is amazed to find her great-grandson David there (his framed photograph), and that "he won't stop looking and smiling at me." Her final word on the day: "That was a real treat!"

June 26   Last week Mom spent days grieving over Dad's death. Today she is angry at him for not looking at her.

"It's not his fault," I say. "It's the way the photographer took the picture years ago. Dad died, but he loves you and wants to hear what you have to say to him."

"I didn't know your father died. What happened?"

"He had a stroke. You called the ambulance."

Mom ponders this news.

"Is he buried?"

* * * * *

Terry and I have an appointment this afternoon. Mom doesn't want to be left alone. We suggest that she could spend a few hours at Cottonwood, a local Adult Day Care facility. She says, "Yes," then, "No," then, "Yes." Then, "I want to do what you do."

At first I take her to mean that she wants to be like us: to go to work, drive a car, be healthy and part of the everyday flow of society. I believe she recognizes, on some level deeper than conscious mind, these aspects of our lives. And remembers that they were once part of hers.

But this is not it. She doesn't *know* what she wants, except that she wants to be with us. And that she does not want to be "left."

June 27 This morning Wayne stayed with Mom at home and it was my turn to drive here to our mountain cabin for a 24-hour stay. Since last autumn we have taken turns, each receiving from the other the gift of an overnight respite here once every two weeks. A day off each fortnight from the pressures of home and business. Time alone. When I'm here I don't worry about Mom. She's safe with Wayne. Sometimes she's happier with Wayne.

Today I am free. Freedom and flowers surround me. Mountain iris, miner's candles, golden banner, dandelions, sulphurflower, cutleaf daisies, fleabane, an occasional gaillardia, cinquefoil, blue penstemon, lupine. Flowers whose names I diligently learn each spring and summer, forget each winter, learn again the following spring. I have sometimes wondered in this past year whether my forgetfulness is a harbinger of a future like my mother's. But today I do not care. Today I am my mother's daughter in another way, a student not of these flowers' names and lineages, but of their beauty.

I have the rest of the day, the uninterrupted night, and tomorrow morning ahead of me, but already I resent the necessary return. Time here by myself is vital to my well-being, to my survival. I would suffocate without it.

The challenge is, can I fulfill my life and help care for my mother? Help her fulfill hers?

June 28 Mom was entirely—and uncharacteristically—relaxed about Terry's departure and absence yesterday, and our interactions throughout the day were some of the most normal I have experienced with her these past eleven months.

When she greets me at her door this morning, however, her face is grim and tight. "I have to feed my husband," she says, her voice a mix of urgency and despair. My anxiety level rises immediately, but what follows is a long and poignant conversation about his death, and her lack of memory of it. Today, at least, she seems to understand the difference between her prized photograph of Russ—"I know this is just a picture," she says—and him. But she clearly does not remember, or perhaps truly believe when I tell her, that he is dead. Our sharing ranges from specific facts and details about him and each of our relationships with him, to our beliefs about death and the possibility of life after death. She caresses Russ's photo as we walk through her grief together, and at the end of our journey I am left with a fuller understanding and acceptance of her sorrow, and of her denial of it, too. It has been a deep and meaningful communication, by any standard. What has brought this on, I wonder, with such force and at just this time?

This evening it suddenly occurs to me that this is the anniversary of Russ's birth. Today he would have been eighty.

Mourning is a difficult process for us all. How does one survive news of the death of a beloved spouse, not once, but over and over again?

— 7 —

June 29, Year One   In one form or another Perry Como has been important to my mother for a very long time. She often told me the story about how she "almost met him." She and my father were at a St. Louis area night club when they spotted him, alone at a nearby table. They wanted to invite him to share their table, or at least they wanted to say hello, but they were too shy.

She was a fan even then, and has remained one these nearly sixty years since. In recent years she became enamored of one particular recording by Mr. Como, "Just Out Of Reach," which she played often—even before she came to Colorado to live. When we visited in California she would play it for us. Then she would play it again. And yet again. When we'd call on the phone from Colorado we could hear the faint melody throughout the conversation, her phonograph set for never-ending repeat of the little disk. When she audiotaped letters to us, there was Perry, in the background, serenading us.

After we moved in together we thought it would be nice for Mom, and us too, to have a broader selection of Perry Como songs to choose from, and so we bought several cassette tapes. During daylight hours our house and vehicles have been a nonstop Perry Como concert ever since.

We think now that "Just Out Of Reach," the song that started it all off, represents my father to her, he himself somewhere beyond her reach for more than two decades now. We've begun to understand that she's very lonely and wants companionship, male companionship especially.

Then came the *Perry Como's Irish Christmas* video, and the image on the front of the box became a person to her. She developed a relationship with him. He, Perry Como, was alive; her husband was dead. Perry Como was within reach; my father was not. The relationship began to take over her life and, by extension, ours as well.

Mom comes out of her room, concerned that her tape isn't playing, and asks for help. I go in and, as is the case more often than not, the tape *is* playing. "It's playing," I say.

"It is not. That's not Perry Como," she says, although she's probably heard this particular tape a hundred times. "I want *Pure Gold*," she says.

I take the cassette out of the player and show her that *Pure Gold* is, in fact, playing (dammit!), although now, of course, it is not.

"That's not it," she says. She brings the empty *Pure Gold* tape box over to me to prove her point. "I want to play *this*."

Sometimes I am wise enough to say pleasantly, "I'll take care of it for you." Then I simply walk in, pop out whatever tape is playing, turn it over, and press the PLAY button. When I do, she is happy, and so am I.

It may be that these requests of hers are not what they seem. It may be that they are attempts at interaction with us. Maybe she just wants to take a few moments to get out of her room, to say a little something, to change the scenery, to reassure herself that we are there, that the world is, if unintelligible, a relatively safe place at least. Maybe she wants to see if her words have an effect, if they result in an action on the part of someone else.

Nevertheless, Mom's efforts to involve us in her reality are an ongoing difficulty for us, and one which continues to escalate.

Not least among her confusions is just who "he" really is—even in *her* mind—for she continues to add new identities to her list: "the sailor," "the doctor," "the young Perry Como," "the real Perry

Como," "Perry Como's son," and even "of all the Perry Comos, this is my favorite."

She talks to him, tells him that she loves him, kisses him. She puts the picture by her pillow, lies on the bed with it and whispers to it, tells it her complaints and the things that have happened or that she has imagined in her day.

Like any relationship, hers with Perry ebbs and flows. She gets mad at him sometimes. She has come out of her room in the evening and demanded to know, "Who is going to take this guy home?" Other times she just wants him "out of there." But when we offer to take him out of there she won't let us. "What are you going to do with him?" she asks protectively. Sometimes, still clinging stubbornly to the "right" reality, we tell her, "We're going to put him on the shelf, along with the other tapes and records," resisting simpler, more agreeable responses along the lines of "We'll take him home," or "We'll see him to the bus." There was a bit of dialogue on TV once about giving someone a ride home. "Boy," Mom lamented, "everybody gets a ride home but my guy."

Sometimes Wayne and I think we should laugh more about this, at least to ourselves, but after eight or ten months the joke has lost its punch. Mom gets into very black moods because of the way her guy is being treated, and how *she* is being treated, insofar as we aren't honoring her requests and her reality. "There's no place set for him at the table. That's no way to treat a guest," she complains. "I love him," she tells us, and real tears roll down her face.

In the beginning we objected to her reality, in a friendly sort of way. "This is just a box," we pointed out. We made jokes. "How much can he eat?" we'd ask, then turn the photograph edge on. "Look how thin he is." Once Wayne sang, "He's only a paper crooner" to the tune of "It's only a paper moon." Sometimes she took these playful comments in good humor, sometimes not. But it didn't matter. More and more her reality took on a life of its own. The fact that we refused to participate in it, and from time to time to refute it, was a frequent source of friction.

One evening, after yet another big argument on the subject, we explained that this is her belief, that this is what she sees. "But it doesn't look that way to us," I told her. "We don't see this as a person. You do, that's okay. But we don't, and so we can't help you with feeding and travel arrangements, where he's going to sleep, and what your relation is with him day to day and hour to hour." I acknowledged her affection and love for him and expressed acceptance of that, but told her that she had to handle those things herself. "My relationship is with you. You have a relationship with me and with him, but I don't have a relationship with him. I have a relationship with you."

I feared that what I was saying was too abstract, too rejecting, or just too long, but it seemed to have a positive impact and things settled down. Feedings at the table ceased. For a while.

Then came a day when she mistook a bit of coloration in the photo on the Perry Como video box as an indication that something was wrong with his face, that he was sick. She wanted to help, and started scraping on it with a scissors. Soon, she had scraped a hole in the face and taken off some of the coloring around the mouth. It upset her, and she wanted me to fix it. I tried to repair the damaged area by working at it with color pencils, but it was hopeless. There was already a hole, and the more I tried to color around it the more the hole grew. "This is the best we can do," I said. "If we try harder it will get worse." Later, I found Mom scratching at it with her nail file. "That's going to make it worse," I cautioned again.

"I think it's making it better," she said.

And so it became a bigger hole, and after a few more days of her ministrations, bigger still, which disturbed her further. At first, when it was just a little mess, she wanted him to go to a barber. When it got worse, she wanted him to go to a doctor. Wayne and I agonized over what to do, and actually gave serious thought to taking her and the box to the doctor. We got caught up in this obsessed, convoluted thinking for days. We were very stressed out about it. Mom was upset, too, if not with us for not taking him, then with him because he refused to go. Then she said he *would* go, but she didn't have a car and couldn't take him. She was crying.

"Okay," I told her, "we'll call the doctor in the morning." And then I worried about *that* all night.

The next morning she didn't mention anything about the doctor. I told her the whole story then, the real story, about how she came to have this picture to begin with. I didn't think it would help. I did it for my sake, for my sanity. I showed her the *Perry Como's Irish Christmas* videotape and how it fit into what was left of the box. I showed her the sales receipt. Everything. "We could do it again," I told her. "We could order a new video and it will come in a new box, with a new picture."

Mom thought this was a great idea. We ordered a new video. Thinking of the long term, Wayne somehow managed on the telephone to convey to the salesperson that the video *box* was an extremely important aspect of the purchase for this particular customer, and the salesperson agreed to (and did) send two extra boxes.

After the new order was placed, Mom was closer than ever with the damaged box. She lay on the bed and held it on her chest with her arms around it. She carried it around all day, took it in the car on trips to the store, holding the picture up and slowly turning it so he could see all the sights as we drove along. She brought it to the dinner table and attempted to feed him in the way that she had so many times before. And, lo and behold, she found that now she could do so!

The meal quickly became an orgy—tuna salad, bread, noodles, green beans—perhaps a third of Mom's plateful went into the box through the hole in the face. Apple juice was next.

"Mom," we protested, "that's just going to pour out onto your lap, onto the floor."

"Let it pour out!" she cried jubilantly. She was thrilled, too thrilled to worry about such petty details.

After dinner she volunteered to bring in a chair from the back yard. This was very unusual, her taking on that kind of task. Not surprisingly, she took the box with her. Wayne watched from the window, both curious and concerned about what she was going to do with this box full of food. Was this going to cause a new confrontation? Because we weren't about to have a box full of rotting food being carried all over the house.

Mom retrieved the chair, folded it, then went over to the fence and picked a single flower, a bachelor's-button. She moved out of Wayne's line of vision then, but came in a minute later. We heard a *thump* in the kitchen. When we had a chance to look we found that the flower she had picked was planted in the picture's mouth, the blossom protruding, the whole thing in the wastebasket.

Today, more than two weeks after the wastebasket incident, Mom writes on a post card to a friend from her old neighborhood in St. Louis: "I am staying at Terry's house. They have room for me and I have a large snapshot of Russ, who I still miss. It is beautiful here, and Russ is here with me. I still miss my Russell, and I have a big snapshot of him."

Despite her confusion—sometimes thinking my father is here, sometimes understanding that she has a snapshot of him—both Wayne and I have found this to be a welcome change from her obsession with the box. Dealing with sadness over her husband's death, even by talking to and kissing and licking his photograph, seems healthier than lavishing the same attentions on a video box cover. She seems more present with us of late, out of her room more, talking and spending time with us. Today she allowed me to give her her vitamins and thyroid medication in her room, something she never permitted previously, because of the various guys.

Wayne and I are reminded again and again that nothing is static with Mom. She changes from day to day. We never know what is coming. We struggle daily to find that difficult balance between honoring and loving her unconditionally on the one hand, and honoring ourselves and our lives on the other. Perhaps the answer lies not in finding some elusive balance, but in learning that love is not a balancing act in the first place.

If you want anything from anyone, you cannot love them fully,
because they are still being weighed in the balance . . .
                                                —Stephen Levine

June 30, Year One I can't figure it all out yet. I can't figure
out unconditional love. I'm used to loving Wayne and Mom *because*
they're Wayne and Mom. Now I'm thinking that I've got to learn
to love her (and Wayne, too) just because she's here. Because she *is*,
and not for any relationship I have or had with her. I have to love
her no matter what happens, no matter how she is now or how she
changes.

July 1 This evening we've joined a group of friends at Christy and
Zander's house for dinner. My mother has been included, as she has
been from the day she came to live with us. She enjoys watching the
children and converses a little with the adults, hampered though she
is by her disease. Her favorite member of the easy-going group is
Paul Newman. He shows up when the bottle of dressing is placed on
the counter next to the salad. She's thrilled to see him. A familiar
face in a crowd is always welcome.

On the way out, Mom says goodbye to Christy and Zander, and
then skips off to the kitchen to bid a reluctant farewell to Paul.

July 3 Mom is quite involved with my dad's photo today. "I
picked him up and put him in bed," she tells us. "I showed him
where the bathroom is." Later, she says, "My friend's in there,"
pointing first to Dad's picture, then to the closed bathroom door.

Wayne says, only half joking, that he fears we are entering a new era, one in which our sole bathroom is regularly commandeered by someone invisible. And with whom it might be difficult to reason.

4ᵗʰ of July   I return from an hour touring the holiday festivities in the park to find Mom and Terry, who have been cat-sitting and watching a movie at Christy and Zander's, in the aftermath of some sort of argument. For a few minutes I am something of a distraction and a leavening influence—until I bring Mom's shoes to her, not at her request.

"I don't want these damn things," she says.

Immediately righteous and indignant, I snarl in her face, "Okay, fine," and proceed to throw her shoes out the door and into the yard. Lamenting their expense, she orders me to go get them.

"*You* go get them," I respond, schoolyard fashion.

Another pair of like exchanges—bitter, yet comical just as surely—and I suddenly relent, retrieve her shoes, and present them to her with what I think a disarming smile. Mom yanks the shoes from my hand, her face disfigured by hurt and fear.

For the moment I am no longer her loved and trusted son-in-law. I am a big, dangerous, mean man.

July 6   My mother frequently writes to my father and "sends" photos to him. She's waiting for him, and angry because he doesn't come or write back. "He would if he could," I tell her. "He loved you so much."

July 10   I borrow the newspaper from my mother-in-law's room. She gives it up easily, but reminds me twice to bring it back.

Fifteen minutes later I return. "Here's your paper," I say with a smile, playfully showing her that I have kept my word.

"I don't want that," she says flatly.

"Okay," I say, in a matter-of-fact tone. I can see her mood has turned surly.

"Nobody told me Terry was going to be gone to the cabin for days."

"Not days," I say quickly—too quickly to dull the retaliatory barb in my tone. I squelch it and continue: "One day. Just one night. She'll be back tomorrow for lunch." I look at the clock: 11:45. "Do you want some lunch?" I ask.

"What?"

"Are you hungry? It's almost lunch time."

"No," she says tersely. "I'll fix my own."

I know that she will not. With the exception of the ill-fated warming of the pie, Mom hasn't once prepared food for herself in over eleven months.

Angry? Or simply not hungry. There is no way for me to know, but I have learned through a year of trial and error that Mom often responds differently if a request, invitation, or suggestion is simply repeated a short while later. Wording is not critical. The trick is to restate with the rhythm, inflection, and body language of an original statement, and to avoid the judgment and impatience that so often overwhelm the message when one feels compelled to repeat. I have found this approach to be dramatically more productive than confrontation and analysis. Mom may not always be able to correctly interpret or express herself in words, but she is uncannily accurate in reading non-verbal messages.

Although I am not always wise and loving enough to choose or even remember this gentler course, today is a good day and thirty minutes later I try again. "Mom, I'm going to make myself some lunch. Do you want me to fix you anything?"

"Yeah. Whatever you're going to have." Smiling, relaxed.

"Oh, just a sandwich probably. I'm not too fancy."

"That sounds fine, Wayne."

July 11   I daydream that my mother gets so well that she sells her car and trailer in California and stays to live on her own in the house on Clevedon. Wayne and I stay with her when we're in town. May this dream come true. This, or something better.

July 16   Mom has found Dad's grave number, which she wrote in her address book long ago. "Look," she says, pointing to the notation.

"Do you know what that is?" I ask.

"Sure. That's where they were supposed to bury him. But they didn't." She cries, then fights against me telling her yet again that Dad is dead. "If he comes back tomorrow, I'll take him back," she tells me.

Should she face the truth, or should I let her think that he might come back at any time? What is the truth, anyway, and what do I know about it? Is Dad "dead"? What does that mean? Does he exist somehow, somewhere, right now? He certainly exists in my mother's mind. Is that delusion, or reality?

Does it matter?

August 7, Year Two   For several days Mom has repeatedly been getting her things together to leave. After a year of living with Wayne and me she continues to view our situation as temporary, herself as a guest in our house. She gathers her essentials—her video, a few audiotapes, a pillow from her bed, two or three random pieces of clothing, her near-empty purse—into a pile on her bed and shows them to me.

"Oh, Mom, don't go," I say each time. "Stay here."

And each time she is relieved. "Good," she says. "I don't want to go."

"You're not," I reassure her.

"I'm glad."

August 12   "Do you remember when we used to chill watermelon in the spring down by the ballfield, and eat it after the game?" my mother asks.

This was something that Mom did when she was an adolescent. So what just happened here? Did I become my mother's childhood friend? Did I become her mother? Or did she simply slip back in time, maintaining her relationship with me as her daughter, but employing some new logic which allows us to exist together in a time before I was born?

August 25 Today is my sister's birthday. When she calls, Mom shares a unique bit of birthday wisdom with her elder daughter. "We all get older if we live long enough," she tells her.

September 2 "Terry, let's go!" Mom demands. Where she wants to go is shopping. I remind her that we have just returned home from shopping. "I don't remember," she says. "Do you know why?" Before I can answer she says, "Don't tell me."

It has been a day also of constant demands by Mom to treat her latest Perry Como picture—this one is from an audiotape box—as a person. "Set a place for him," she says one minute, and "I don't want him in my room" or, just as likely, "Where's my guy?" the next. And now, this evening, she continues: "Can't you take him home? It's dark." She says this over and over. I can't stand it anymore. "Find another place to live," I explode. "Or *you* live here. Wayne and I will move out!"

We are both upset. I leave the room, eventually cool down, then feel remorse about my outburst. How is it that the pain of the argument always seems to exceed the pain that led to the argument?

Although I feel that she treated me unfairly, I know that she can't help it. And I know that I have treated her unfairly, because I can help it. I feel a surge of love, a sure knowledge that our relationship is much deeper than these hassles of the immediate moment.

I go to her room. "We'll work things out, Mom," I tell her, "because we love each other."

"I know," she says.

Maybe I should respond to her unreasonable demands as if they are the antics of a crazy person. Maybe it would keep me from blowing up. Yet sometimes she behaves like a perfectly normal person. Sometimes we meet in the hallway in the middle of the night and she asks me if I'm all right. Sometimes she still acts like my mother.

September 9   I rub my mother's back as strains of "Claire de Lune" drift through the house.

"That feels so good," she says. . . . "Some of the music they play is like rubbing your back."

September 14   My mother has again ruined the face of her guy, this time on the audiotape box, in the same way and for the same reason as previously. Half of the face has been erased by her rubbing, kissing, and licking.

Mom interprets this as his having disappeared. I tell her that we could perhaps find another tape at the music store. Fine. But she wants to go NOW. She wants her guy back NOW.

September 16   No let up in Mom's compulsion. We have gone to music stores, department stores, drugstores, and grocery stores. I have placed an order at the record store, in hopes that they can find a copy. The fact that we cannot locate a replacement for the damaged tape makes no difference to Mom. No sooner do we return from our latest outing to a record store than she approaches me with her purse slung over her arm and a look of urgency in her eyes.

"Well?" she demands, "I thought we were going."

"Going where?"

"To get my guy!" she exclaims with frustration.

September 22   For a week now, my mother has wanted me, many times each day, to check if the ordered tape has arrived at the store. She wants me to go there, to find him, to bring him home. It's been a week of almost constant argument. "We'll call once a day," we agree, but moments later Mom has forgotten.

Now, once again she insists on going. "Mom, we just called and they don't have it," I say, and refuse to take her.

"Then I'll go on my own," she declares and walks out the door, around the corner and up the street, wending her way through the massive maze of tree branches that lie everywhere, branches brought down in full leaf by an early heavy snowfall.

An hour later she hasn't returned. Wayne searches by car for thirty minutes but comes back alone. We go together, eventually ranging more than a mile east, all the way down to the church, to her favorite supermarket, scouring the side streets to no avail until, suddenly, we come upon her three blocks from home. She's been missing for two hours.

September 23   "I wish I could find my other purse!"

"I don't know where it is." What I do know is that my mother has only one purse.

"Because I know that's where that thing would be because I have never taken it out of there. You're sure you don't have it in your room?"

"Don't have what?"

"My other purse in your room."

"No. No, I don't have any of your things in my room."

That "thing" Mom is referring to is her second ruined Perry Como picture. So Wayne takes one of the extra *Irish Christmas* boxes—not so useless after all, it seems—laminates it at Kinko's, and gives it to Mom. She tapes it on her wall, then removes it and carries it around the house, thrilled to have it again.

But, she's still looking for her *other* guy.

September 25   Sharon calls each week to talk to Mom, and to us about how Mom is doing. Today Wayne brings up the subject of her and Denny taking care of Mom out there for several weeks this fall. Sharon thinks it would be really hard. "To tell you the truth," she says, "I don't know if we can do it," and adds, "I think you must be saints." Wayne tells her, "She needs to be with someone. And we have to have some times to do our work. We need some breaks." Sharon says they will give it a try.

I can see that they would have a problem. I understand that it's very hard for them. Part of it is just logistics, like David having to move into another room. That's very hard. And then there are all the other family dynamics. I can see all that, and it bothers me. I don't want to make their lives harder but, like Wayne, I want their help.

I can also imagine that Mom might not have much of a good time out there after the first few days or even hours. She'll have done her visiting and will want to come home here to her own bed and familiar surroundings, as though they are around the corner. And that bothers me, for all their sakes.

Wayne tells me that Sharon told him at one point, "Oh, I understand. Believe me, I understand that you need that time." And he felt that it was a sincere statement. "But I don't want to be declared a saint," he tells me. "I want help."

Sharon didn't choose to live with Mom. We did. We can't expect them to fill in for us when we want or need it. From the beginning Sharon felt it was better for Mom to be in a nursing home. That was her preference. We made our own choice.

The bottom line for me is that I don't really know what's best for Mom, don't know if we're doing what's best. I worry that we will make a bad decision, one that can't be undone.

September 26 "What is a saint?" Terry asks, as if I might actually know. "At school we were encouraged to be like them. I read *Lives Of The Saints*. I wanted to be one. And now several people in the past year have called us saints. But what is a saint?"

"I only know that it has something to do with hiding the Blessed Sacrament under your coat," I tell her, "and not letting on, even though wolves may claw your skin. Hmmm. Come to think of it, this past year has been something like that. Maybe we *are* saints!"

"I think you're mixing up saints and Spartans," she says.

"Really? Well, we're becoming one or the other!"

September 27 "Shit!"

The word rings out from my mother-in-law's bedroom as she searches for her blue comb for what must be the tenth time this morning. We've been singing the Blue Comb Blues this past week or so. She looks for her comb, off and on, all day. Sometimes she holds it in her hand as she asks us where it might be. It sounds funny. And sometimes, when we're not too exhausted, we laugh.

I hear Mom's footsteps in the hallway and know what is coming. "Have you seen my blue comb?" she asks.

Not for several minutes, I think as I step into her bedroom and quickly spot the perfect outline of her comb between the pillow and the pillowcase. "What is this?" I tease.

"That's my blue comb," she says as if nothing could be of less interest to her.

September 28   While she eats her dinner, Mom gazes at her framed photo of my father, which she clutches.

"You'd really like to see Dad," I venture.

"Yeah. Just like I would be gla-a-ha"—she stutters, uncharacteristically stumbles on the simple word before substituting another—"*happy* to see Sharon."

"I know."

"She sends me pictures of her and all the kids. She sent me some today."

"Today?" Wayne asks.

"Yeah."

"Well, those are pictures that you've had," I explain. "I found them again and gave them to you yesterday, but Sharon sent them a while ago."

"Oh," Mom says. Somehow Wayne and I have veered once more onto the path of Truth. As though it's important for Mom to know that the pictures didn't come today. She blows on her chili, takes a spoonful into her mouth. Dad looks on. "When did you find those things in my wallet?"

"Well, they were in your wallet. And then you took them out, and now you found them again. You used to always keep them in your wallet."

Again my answer is longer than Mom needs. By the time I finish she has turned her attention to the framed, age-yellowed photograph in her left hand. "He's smiling," she says, pointing at the sepia lips with her spoon. "Makes you feel he'd like to come."

"Well, he's here in spirit," Wayne offers.

"I wonder if he's still a meat cutter," Mom muses. . . . "I wish he would come."

"If he could come he would," I say, "but he's here in spirit."

"What do you mean?" she asks. "He's dead?" Without waiting for an answer she kisses his picture, then looks up, looks at me. "I wouldn't even know where to write him," she laments. "I don't think he's working in the store anymore." She's referring to a neighborhood grocery store my dad and his brother owned until the late '50's. For the rest of his life he was a meat cutter in a supermarket. Mom has forgotten that, too.

September 29   After a rainstorm this evening Mom calls me into her room. "Look at the rainbow! Look at all the colors!" She loves to see the sky's different lights—morning and evening, sunrises, the moon, the stars, rainbows.

This very morning there was a rare rainbow in the west. Mom and Wayne and I all went out to look at it, stood there on the dew-dampened lawn in our bathrobes before 7 a.m., admiring.

— 9 —

"There's a man in my bed!"
—Helen

October 1, Year Two   We receive from the printer advance copies of our new book, *Night Of The Falling Stars*. Mom says to me, "Your father should see you. He'd be so proud. He always wanted to write." It is a tender, shared memory, but Mom is soon distracted. "There's a red dog," she says, pointing out the window.

October 3   My mother-in-law and I arrive at the post office on this beautiful Indian Summer day and park in the usual lot.

"Do you want to come in with me?" I ask, and she answers as I expect, that she prefers to stay in the car, listening to her music.

But before I am fully out of the vehicle she asks, "Don't you have any windows in this car?"

Her question throws me. Like most cars, our Subaru wagon is encircled by a virtual ribbon of glass. It takes me a moment to realize that she is simply too warm and that, although the window crank is inches from her hand, she doesn't know how to operate it, doesn't even know that it exists.

I hadn't realized: the car that *Mom* is in has no windows at all.

October 5   "Terry. I need you."

I find Mom in the bathroom, pulling her slacks on over her pajama bottoms. She knows that something is wrong but she doesn't know what it is, or how to fix it.

Afterward, she goes into her room. I hear the muted protest of aged springs as she sits on the edge of her bed. "They've got all my clothes here to convince me that I live here," she confides to imaginary friends, "but I don't."

Mom's floor is sticky. Apple juice stains run down the wall below the picture of Perry Como. We show this to her, tell her not to feed him because it's not good for the wall and floor.

"Okay," she agrees, "but things are pretty confusing around here."

October 6   A knock on our door in the middle of another too-short night. "Are you there, Terry?" she calls through the wood.

"Mom, it's two o'clock."

"The cars are outside. I just wondered if you were here."

Wayne has left early for a day and night of respite at the cabin. Alone now in the quiet morning kitchen I see that Mom had cookies and made coffee during the night. She didn't use the hot water in the Thermos we've made ready for her each day. She used all the instant coffee in the jar and mixed it in a glass of tap water. Not surprisingly, the viscous brown drink sits here on the counter still.

"Mom, did you have a restless night?" I ask when she comes searching for me and breakfast.

"I've been pushing these things in my head all the time," she says angrily. "Oh, I've 'gotta have someone with me all the time.'" She rattles the words off like a sarcastic teen. "Which is a lot of bullshit."

Did she hear this somewhere? From us? Has she pulled it from some time-out-of-mind memory of the Diagnosis Meeting at the hospital over a year ago?

Mom wants to go and look for her guy. I wear myself out arguing with her, but she wants to look for him no matter what I say. I tell her I won't go with her and she says she'll go look for him herself, and that she doesn't care if she gets lost. "If you don't care if you'll get lost then you are sick, Mom, because that's sick to not care if you're going to get lost," I tell her.

Oh, that's very good. Really brilliant.

My friend Jean drops by and I persuade her to stay for dinner. Mom argues that if I'm going to have my friend to dinner she should be able to have her friend. "But there's no place for him," she says pointedly.

"Bring him in," I tell her. "I'll make sure there's a place for him."

She goes to her room, comes back empty-handed, sits down at her place. I look at her, raise my eyebrows in a wordless question.

"I couldn't carry him," she explains.

Jean should visit more often. Mom and I have both improved our behavior. Or at least our manners.

October 7   By 3:30 Terry has Mom dressed and ready for me to take her to church for the 4 p.m. Mass. In her lap she holds her envelope for the collection basket, sealed and marked "$2.50." I note that this constitutes a sudden and generous 25% increase over her offerings of the past year. Ah! But something less benign is afoot: her envelope is lumpy. Perhaps a popcorn offering?

My nimble fingers soon determine that it is neither popcorn nor $2.50 inside the envelope, but Mom's rosary. This seems a crisis of some import, as Mom's purple rosary is the last remaining arti-cle—if you don't count crumpled tissues—residing regularly in her purse.

I quickly find another envelope and two dollar bills and present them to Mom. She inserts the bills, seals the envelope and hands it back to me.

"You give it," she says. "I have my own."

I try by some sleight of hand to substitute one envelope for the other but, proving that while her mind may be slowing down her eye is still faster than my hand, she informs me, "This isn't mine. There's nothing in this one."

"There is," I insist truthfully. "There's two dollars." Mom doesn't buy it. She believes in a lumpy envelope.

At Mass, the service rushes toward the Offertory and I busy myself with devising a plan to rescue Mom's sacrificial rosary. Finally, even as the ushers begin rattling their wicker sabers, I hit upon an ingenious solution.

"Mom," I whisper, "your rosary is inside your envelope."

She looks at me with amazement—terror even—in her eyes, rips it open immediately, and rescues the beads. "Oh, my God!" she exclaims reverently. Locally, eyes are momentarily diverted from the sanctuary toward us. One never knows when a vision may have occurred.

The usher draws near now, but I am fearless. I congratulate myself, luxuriate in my victory. As the collection basket slips like a well-oiled piston across the laps of the faithful in the pew in front of us Mom takes the cue and reaches into her purse—Wait! What is this she's pulling out? *Another* envelope?

I have forgotten: I gave to Mom less than an hour ago a greeting card from my mother that arrived in today's mail. The basket slides in from my right. I drop the money envelope in. The basket reaches Mom—and she donates my mother's card and letter, still in their unopened envelope! A scant moment later the basket passes by me again, in reverse. I reach in—an unorthodox move—and withdraw my mother's envelope, smiling sweetly at the usher as I do so.

He pauses. Our eyes meet. He decides to cut his losses, withdraws the basket and its remaining contents quickly, and moves on to the next pew. Mom misses the whole thing.

In the end, we go in peace.

October 8 Yesterday my mother was talking about being "transferred" and seemed very concerned. Today, while talking with her about going to Sharon's I explain, "You're going to be there for awhile, and then after you visit with them you'll come back here and we'll have all your stuff here."

She lets out a sigh of relief. "Who are you going to use the room for when I'm not here?" she asks.

"Nobody. We're going to keep it for you."

"Oh, good!"

I think we've solved the transfer problem.

October 10 Mom and Wayne have just returned from shopping. She gets out of the car, slumping with exhaustion. He comes up beside her and puts his arm around her. She gives a big sigh.

I can't count the times I've seen this or scenes like it. I never tire of them.

October 11 Wayne and I have decided we need a day together in the mountains, hiking through golden aspen. I've packed a picnic lunch. We *need* to go. But I am both worried and guilt-ridden about leaving my mother alone.

"Mom, will you be okay by yourself all day?"

"No, I'll kill somebody."

"We'll be home in time for dinner. I'm not worried about you killing anybody. I just wondered if you're going to be okay."

"Of course."

"I've got your lunch all made and I'm going to put it in the refrigerator."

"Put it where that guy can't get to it."

"You know where the cookies are, right? Up in the cupboard?"

"No."

"Well, look—"

"Oh. The box of cookies?"

"Yeah, the box of cookies is up here in the cupboard."

"Okay. . . . And I'm going to go for a walk."

"Okay."

"I'm going to find my guy if it's the last thing I do."

The three of us get into a ten minute harangue. Finally, Wayne and I extract a "promise" from Mom that she won't go looking for her guy. Good enough. We're going.

Really worried. Really guilt-ridden. But going.

When we get home Wayne and I are relieved to find Mom safe and sound, but I am hardly across the threshold before she starts clamoring for me to take her places to find her guy again. She wants to "induct him into a small hospital," she says, or "find him at the drugstore."

* * * * *

"Terry, there's a man in my bed!" Mom's urgent whisper pushes through our bedroom door. It's dark, and I'm tired, and it's the middle of the night. I'm glad it's Terry Mom is asking for.

"No, no, Mom," she says. "There's no one. Go back to bed."

"Yes! I can see him. I want you to get him out."

Terry gets up and follows Mom to her room. In the dark I hear a ruffling of bed clothes next door. Perhaps he is putting up a fight.

"What are you going to do with him?" I hear Mom ask with as much concern as curiosity.

"Wayne will take care of it," Terry says, her own tone leaving no room for doubt.

The door hinge creaks, a shaft of light slices across the room.

"Okay," Mom agrees.

Terry's hand and arm slip through the narrow opening, flex once, and a fluttery, boomerang sort of noise fills the room for a moment—and then the laminated Perry Como "trespasser" caroms off my head.

October 12 "Terry, let's go get my guy," Mom says.

"Not now, Mom," I answer, trying to figure out what to make for supper.

She walks out the door, angry. An hour goes by. I have the feeling that she's really gone again, just like three weeks ago. After an hour and a half of driving I find her, standing on the side of the road, wild-eyed, clutching the cover of the Perry Como record album that I got for her a couple of days ago. Tonight she threatens to walk off again.

I'm exhausted. I can't bear these hassles over wanting me to go and find something I can't find, or to take her someplace where she can't find it, either. My life has become a single scene, a tape loop that plays over and over. Endlessly.

October 16 I unexpectedly run into our friend Jeb at the post office. He lived with and took care of his father for years before the older man's death from Alzheimer's three years ago. I tell Jeb about the turmoil Wayne and I are experiencing with my mother. "Just love her," he tells me.

October 17 I put a new Bing Crosby tape on for my mother. The mere fact that it is a change from Perry Como energizes me and I start dancing around the house.

"Are you going nuts?" Mom wants to know.

"Probably."

"I *am* nuts," she says.

October 18 Wayne loads Mom's suitcase in the back of the car. "Where do I tell them I'm going?" she asks me as we watch from the doorway.

"Wayne knows. He'll take care of it for you. You just relax, Mom."

We walk the few yards from door to curb. "You'll tell me when it's time to come back here," she says, half statement, half question.

"I will," I promise.

Seven o'clock.

I sit in twilight thinking of Mom, picturing her on the plane. Without Wayne. Without me. Hanging there in the air, chasing the too-fast sun alone. "Where do I tell them I'm going?" she asked me. Where indeed?

It's seven o'clock, and I'm crying.

— 10 —

How dull it is to pause, to make an end,
To rust unbumished, not to shine in use!
                    —Alfred Lord Tennyson,
                      "Ulysses"

"I can't stay with you forever. I can't be around your neck."
                    —Helen

October 19, Year Two   I woke often last night, moaning and groaning loudly, aches and pains and sadness escaping from me like steam from a pressure cooker. This morning I feel lighter, healthier, though worried already about the time when Mom will return. I love the freedom. It's like getting out of prison.

Sharon calls. "Things aren't going well," she says. "She's feeling abandoned. She wants to come back. She's packed her suitcase twice."

When Mom gets on the phone she is upset, although I've heard her a lot worse. Her opinion is that she's been there for three or four days already. She is done with visiting and wants to come back. That's the big theme: "When are you going to come and get me?"

"You're going to come on the plane. It'll be a couple of weeks."

"Okay. . . . *When* are you going to come now? Should I drive up there?"

October 27   "Sharon won't let me go anywhere," Mom complains. She sounds down.

"Where do you want to go?"

"I want to go out."

"With whom, Mom?"

"With Perry Como. . . . I'm an adult, but they're treating me like I'm a kid. What am I, a teenager? I want to go out." She sounds like a very young, petulant, Perry Como groupie. But she knows that she is an adult, and takes umbrage at having to ask permission to go out. Perfectly logical. "Remember," she tells me, "you're my daughter. If I can't go out, you can't either." Well, sort of logical.

"Sharon just wants you to be safe," Wayne says. "It's dark out, and she doesn't want you to—"

"It'd be okay, I'd be with this guy."

"Where do you want to go?" he asks.

"To the show."

"How would you get there?"

"In a car."

"Whose car?"

"We've got a couple of guys who have cars," Mom assures him.

"Okay," I say, "when they come in their car and pick you up, then you can go."

"Good."

October 31   After twelve days apart, I'm starting to let go of my intense involvement with my mother and relax into my own life, finally getting the relief I need in order to be able to take her back.

November 1   "I won't be coming today, Terry. Or tomorrow."

"Okay."

"To your house. . . . Because I have found something out."

"What, Mom?"

"I'm at Sharon's."

November 7   Wayne and I have checked out the Secure Alzheimer's Unit at a local nursing home, talked to the social worker, and filled out an application form. No obligation. And no urgent need. But there is smoke in the wind. It seems the prudent thing to do.

Earlier, we stopped by Park Street Senior Day Care and signed Mom up for next Thursday morning. She'll be home by then, and we have a business appointment that day in Boulder.

Sharon and I talk a long time about non-resuscitation orders, nursing homes, Medicaid, the car title. Not long after we hang up she calls back to say that she has just returned from searching for Mom. While Sharon and I were on the phone, Mom walked out the door and covered nearly half a mile before they found her. She told Sharon she was looking for our house. We talk about whether Mom is going to be a wanderer. I don't know, but I do know this: when my mother wants something, she wants it. She's not a passive person.

Nor, come to think of it, do I believe that "wanderer" is an apt word. Wandering suggests aimless movement, with no plan or destination. Mom always has a plan and a destination—to find us, our house, her mobile home, her guy. She may have been mistaken today about where our house is, but she was not wandering.

November 8 I wait at the United gate, peering down the flimsy-looking corridor that births the sky-world people back to the ground. As I watch, it spews out passengers fitfully, singly and in small knots. A fellow in a business suit passes close, pauses a moment, eyeing me.

"Are you waiting for your mother?" he asks.

"Yes. My mother-in-law," I answer, somehow pleased with his erroneous presumption. More than anything, though, I am startled by the fact that he has addressed me at all.

"She's coming," he says. "She's fine."

He moves toward the escalator, leaving me uneasy in his wake, all the more so for his reassurances. I pace, adjusting my angle as though to see around impenetrable corners, to locate my fine mother in the belly of the plane. Moments later another man emerges from the grey passage. He, too, speaks to me unsolicited, and in almost the same words as his predecessor. I follow him a few steps, even as I catch a glimpse of Mom now at the far end of the tube.

"Is everything okay?" I ask. "Is there a problem?"

"Oh, no." He smiles pleasantly. "No, there's no problem."

No problem. But it is clear that at least two passengers on this airplane know who Mom is. And that somebody must be waiting for her. For that matter, I can only guess what *I* must look like, to be so accurately identified, twice, amidst the throng of eager greeters in one of the busiest airports in the nation!

Mom strides toward me now, with good energy, a brisk step and a smile and a wave. I smile and wave, too, all the while busily scanning her for telltale signs. Of what, I have no idea.

She *looks* okay. We hug. She *feels* okay.

"I told a man," she promptly and happily informs me, "that I left my green suitcase here a couple of days ago. He told me, 'We're keeping it for you.' "

"And I know just where it is, Mom. Let's go get it."

She has indeed flown friendly skies. For the moment at least, it feels like the whole world has taken her under its wing.

November 9   Having dropped my mother off at Park Street Senior Day Care this morning as planned, Wayne and I return at 2 p.m. Mom explodes out the door and meets us on the run, a young lady that we've never seen before trailing after her.

"They wouldn't let me go outside. They were pushing me and pulling at me. They were showing dirty movies." Her words rush out in a continuous string. She is panting.

"Mom, hold on," I say. "Calm down. Everything's okay."

"Where is Terry?" she says to me. "Is Terry at home?"

"Mom, *I'm* Terry," I answer, unable to hide my surprise.

"No, you're not," she scoffs. "Where's Wayne's wife?"

November 10 Terry's dream:

A holiday gathering, Thanksgiving maybe, a table laden with food. Mom is here, and Wayne, and other people that I know, family and friends. Mom says to me, "What did your dad say before he went to hell?"

"Dad didn't go to hell," I protest.

She giggles like a little girl. "Where did he go then?"

"Heaven."

Suddenly Dad is there, sitting in the chair next to her. My heart leaps with surprise and happiness and I go over to him, just to be near. His hand is on my head now, a fatherly caress. I want childhood back, my dad to take care of me. To take care of everything.

"Can't you stay with us and help us?" I plead.

"No," he says, even as he starts to fade . . .

November 12 "I hate to leave him," my mother tells me through sudden tears, clutching her picture of Perry Como to her chest.

"You don't have to leave him," I tell her. "You can stay here. Where do you think you're going?"

"To a nursing home."

I am shocked to hear these words from her lips; thrown completely off balance. Not because they are unreal, but because they seem, some days at least, so very real, so close. I have been hiding them in my head, or so I believed, and I can hardly bear to hear her speak them.

"Why do you say that?" I ask.

She answers without hesitation; with grief, but without tears. "Because I don't have any home."

She's feeling insecure, I tell myself. The day after her return from Sharon's we had her at Park Street. Maybe she perceived, or was told, that it was like a nursing home. Wayne and I have been worrying about what to do this spring when we need to travel. Maybe she's overheard snatches of our conversations. Maybe she's trying to figure out a solution for herself. Maybe she can read minds.

"You're staying here with us as long as we have this house." I say the words as though they are an edict.

"I can't stay with you forever," Mom replies. "I can't be around your neck."

November 13 "People were trying to get in the windows!" Mom tells us when we return after leaving her alone in the house for three daylight hours. "I never want to be alone again!" Wayne uses this as an opportunity to offer Cottonwood Adult Day Care—which Mom tried for one day last summer and didn't like—as a place to go when we have to work. "Okay," Mom agrees. "Good."

November 15 Mom went to Cottonwood yesterday, stayed all day and went back again today, albeit with some resistance, complaining that she has "never heard anything about it."

November 16 Today when we arrive at Cottonwood Mom refuses to get out of the car. "I want to go down and see the football game," she says.

Wayne drives to where the team was practicing when we drove by yesterday, and parks in the empty lot. We look out through alternating fog and drizzle at acres of green, empty field.

"Well, here it is," Wayne says. "I don't know why you want to be here."

Mom is tense in front of me, her back pushed against the seat cushion. Is she thinking that we have intentionally taken her to the wrong place? The muscle in Wayne's jaw pulses rhythmically as he stares out into the damp. He's calling her bluff, giving her a chance to do what she said she wanted to do, to see what she has chosen. Logical consequences. Only logical consequences don't work so well with somebody who has dementia. Mom has no idea why we're sitting here.

"Would you get this thing off me!" she demands, fumbling ineffectually with the clasp of her seatbelt.

"No," Wayne says flatly.

She struggles with it, gets it undone, but now can't get her door open. She paws and slaps at the door panel.

"Okay, let's relax," I tell them both, and myself, too. "Take deep breaths. Let's talk this through."

"I'm sorry," Mom says quickly, though in a pouting tone.

"Mom, look. We're a family, aren't we?" Wayne says.

"Of course we're a family."

"Okay. Well, families need to work together. We have things to do, you have things to do."

"I've done that place. I told you that."

"Well, Mom, it's either there or we can sit here in the cold and you can look at this empty field. Your choice."

"Fine."

"Mom," I say, "why don't we go back and see if a staff member could take you for a walk later? Maybe the weather will be nicer then, too."

Long seconds of silence from the front seat. "Let's go check," Mom says.

Back at Cottonwood, a female volunteer we have never met before comes out to greet us. I ask about the possibility of a walk for Mom. "Sure, we could do that," she says, full of youth and smiles.

Mom gets out of the car without urging or assistance and goes in. We leave. I'm exhausted before the day has started.

When we pick her up, Mom's only comment is that we are late. In fact, we are several minutes early, but we understand that her message to us is not about time. We go into the building, hoping to demonstrate to her that we are comfortable here, that the three of us are part of this place, together. Mom doesn't want to go back in, and when she finally does, she lingers near the door. "Look at all those people sleeping in that room," she says. I look where she points: a lazy arc of chairs, and almost every occupant asleep.

At home she is in an excellent mood, speaks positively to us about how they fed her, then repeats the stories to the guys in her room and bursts into song.

I think it may be the best afternoon I've seen her have in these nearly sixteen months. I really feel that this is going to work out.

November 17 This morning we pull into the Cottonwood lot and as soon as Mom sees the building she says, "You're not going to park *me* here!" My heart drops.

Wayne takes a breath and lets out a long sigh. We have to go to work, he tells her; we need to make money. This is not a bad tack to take. Mom grew up during the Great Depression. As a teenager she had to quit school and take a job cleaning other people's houses. She understands the necessity of money. She goes in without further urging.

At home later, she remarks again on the strangeness of the people there, imitates them by closing her eyes and scrunching up her face and making clonic-like movements of her arms and hands. "They can't talk," she complains.

December 1 "Where's Wayne taking me?" she asks Terry en route to Cottonwood. "Not to that place."

"Well, it's where you go," Terry says. "Where else are we going to take you? We're going to school. That's your school."

Mom's tone changes abruptly. "There's a man there who does his homework," she says as though sharing an interesting slice of campus life.

"See? It's like a school."

"There's one lady who just sleeps." She chuckles.

"Yeah, and you don't," Terry encourages. "You can ask them to play your tapes and . . . do different things there."

Mom asks for the note we always give her, the one which states that we will pick her up at the assigned time; the one which assures her, momentarily at least, that she is not abandoned, that we will return for her. She folds it up, stashes it safely in her empty purse.

We turn onto the patch of asphalt parking area. "Don't tell me we're *here* already!" Mom exclaims, astonished and disappointed.

One of her favorite staff members opens the door, smiles at her. Mom smiles back, gets out of the car, and goes into Cottonwood without apparent emotion, without a word to anyone.

Your school. Our school. This is one of our lies. We don't attend school. And, due in large part to Mom's needs, we have been to schools to make our presentations only rarely in recent months.

Even in those cases, of course, it would be more accurate to say that we were going "to work." Most of what little work we have been able to accomplish—as we hope to do today—has been writing. At home. But we're not about to say "we're going back home."

While we acknowledge Mom's feelings verbally, and honor them in our hearts, the truth is that we do not honor them in our actions. Despite her objections, we do leave her there, and in doing so deny her control over her life yet one more time. What she says, what she wants—more often than not, these things do not change the reality of her life.

The simple fact is that we have to have some relief and assistance if we are going to survive—emotionally, physically, and financially. We believe, too, that Mom needs something and somebody besides us. She seems genuinely to like a couple of the staff at Cottonwood. Sometimes she objects strenuously to going, other times she is eager. We keep bringing her, hoping that the place will somehow "take"; that it will become a regular habit, perhaps even a source of pleasure for her. Even though it doesn't seem the right place, we need something, and Cottonwood is all that we have.

I crave an alternative, so that Mom doesn't have to be by herself—frightened and lonely and bored—and so that Terry and I can have time. Time to be alone. Time to work. Time to breathe.

December 10   As Mom heads out the door with Wayne to go shopping it appears to me that something is amiss. There are great bulges under the back of her sweater.

"Mom, wait a minute. Something's wrong. Let me see," I say, pulling her back from the door. I lift the back of her sweater and am amazed to find that she is wearing not one but two of her prosthetic bras, the second outside her shirt and facing the rear.

"Here, Mom, let's get this off," I say, stifling a laugh as I tug at the sleeves. When she sees what she has done she laughs out loud over it. "Oh, my God!" she exclaims as I remove the back-facing bra, and I laugh, too. She doesn't seem to take things like this too seriously, either as a problem or as anything to be ashamed of.

And, contrary to my impressions of the past quarter century, Wayne is apparently not quite as observant of the details of female anatomy as I thought he was.

December 11   As I usher my mother-in-law through Cottonwood's front door I can't help but see again the young man in a chair to my right. I've seen him here before. Several times.

I call him "young" meaning as I am young, probably in his forties. Too young to be a client here. The first time I saw him I assumed he was a volunteer, on staff, or a Board member. I've seen him several times now. I think he wears a name tag. Like Mom.

I have a hard time relating to him, acknowledging him even. Saying hi to the little old ladies, that's easy. But this man looks too young; his skin is too smooth. I simply don't *want* to believe that he is a client. If not a volunteer, if not on staff, then let him be a visitor, a worker from the crew resurfacing the street outside who has stopped in for a cup of coffee. Anything.

That's what I want, but I think that's not the way it is.

He is at once alert and aware and yet distant and detached. His eyes are all-seeing, but unblinking and vacant, too. Sometimes he seems dead, propped there in the chair; other times I think that he is on guard, has made himself very small and retreated somewhere inside this outer armor. If I touch him, I sometimes wonder, will he ring hollow?

Today I don't even see him at first. It is his movement that catches my eye. He looks up when I greet a staff member.

"Hello," he murmurs from right beside me, his voice meek but startling me just the same.

I smile weakly. "Hello," I say, but go no further.

I don't look him in the eye when I return his greeting. I tell myself that to do so would be to taunt him, as though to say, "I'm coming in from outside and I'll be leaving here in a few seconds. You're going to be here all day."

But that's not it. I do not look in this man's face because I am afraid that if I do the face I see will be mine.

— 11 —

As though to breathe were life! Life piled on life
Were all too little, and of one to me
Little remains . . .

                —Alfred Lord Tennyson,
                  "Ulysses"

December 15, Year Two Some time ago, Cottonwood gave me a Do Not Resuscitate form for my mother. If DNR is our request, they need authorization on file, signed by me and by her physician. Wayne and I have talked about it, agreed on it, and I've signed it. The other day I brought it to Mom's doctor, who looked at it a moment, said, "Oh yeah," and signed it. But now that it's ready to go back to Cottonwood I find myself stuck in some emotional mud. Turning it in formalizes that Mom is sick, so sick that if her heart stops beating no one will try to save her. It means that I don't *want* anyone to try to save her, even if they could bring her back without any further deterioration in her condition or abilities. I wouldn't sign a form like that for Wayne. I don't like making that distinction between two people whom I love.

Wayne reminds me that everybody tells us she's only going to get worse. That she won't know people, that she'll be unhappy all the time, that she'll forget how to eat or swallow. If everybody's right, he says, one day she'll probably need a nursing home. Maybe she'll fall down, break her hip, and die of pneumonia. If she dies before that, let her be. That's all the form says, he tells me.

He's not being uncaring, I know. Fewer clouds of guilt and fear lie between him and this piece of paper, and he's sharing his clearer vision with me in the hope of being helpful.

My problem is that I want this to be my mother's decision, her signature on the form, want at least to be able to talk to her about it. But I can't do that. She doesn't grasp her situation. She's never even acknowledged that she *has* Alzheimer's.

I cannot talk to my mother about the DNR. I cannot.

December 17   For their annual Christmas Open House, our friends April and Anthony have laid out seventeen plates and bowls of homemade goodies. Wonderful cookies of every shape and taste and texture. My mother tries them all. She eats and eats, drinks cold punch and hot cider, and is friendly with everyone. She even sticks out her hand to a stranger, who does not respond in kind. Perturbed but undefeated, she instructs him. "Shake my hand," she says, which he finally does.

She has a wonderful time. When we get home she proclaims, "That was the best meal I ever had."

* * * * *

Just prior to the best meal she ever had I took Mom on one of my little errand trips so that Terry could relax alone. When I returned to the car after one of my stops Mom scolded me for my absence. "I went in there looking for you," she told me, pointing to a toy store—not where I had been—right in front of the car.

I thought maybe she was lying to me, just making up a story and filling in the blank with the store name that was right before her eyes. But I noticed that her seatbelt was unfastened. And her story had some detail. She said that she went in and told a clerk, "I'm looking for my son-in-law," and that they didn't know who she was talking about.

So, I think she *did* get out of the car. It suddenly occurs to me that this is the fourth time in less than a week that she has gotten out of the car. It seems to be her new thing to do.

My first thought is that maybe this is a good sign: she's taking action, asking questions, going for what she wants. But my second thought, the one I'm more inclined to believe, is that she's becoming more impulsive. She doesn't know if it's been three minutes or three hours, and she doesn't care. She's bored, she's tired of waiting, she wants me, she'll go find me. She's not skillful at it. She just walks into whatever building is more or less in front of her, and starts requesting that they produce her son-in-law.

Yesterday, during extra-vehicular excursion #3, she had better success. She got out of the car and went into the library, an accurate guess on her part, although the odds were in her favor as it was the only building on the entire block. She talked to the Children's Librarians, most of whom, as it happens, know Terry and me because of our children's books. I suppose she got them all wondering, *Where's Wayne?* Or perhaps, after a time, something more along the lines of, *Where in the hell is Wayne, anyway?*

I happened to come down the stairs at that moment, saw her talking to them, came over and put my arm around her. "Oh, here he is!" they said, and Mom giggled. Then she slapped me a couple of times on the arm. Kind of punched me. It didn't hurt, but it surprised me and got me thinking about impulsivity for the first time.

Come to think of it, she's been doing things like that with me quite a lot in the past week or two. Poking me in the arm, tapping me on the chin. The other day she jabbed me lightly with her fork. Playful kinds of things, done in a jovial mood, but in the past she would have just pretended. Now the tines have found my skin.

December 18   Once again I've brought my mother to the record store. She wants to look for "the kid." We rummage through the bins: the oldies, the sale stuff, the C's for Como.

I ask the salesperson for assistance. He checks his inventory and confirms what I already know: the kid isn't here. At my request he finds an address to write to for Perry Como recordings, pulls up this information on the computer, swings the monitor to face us so I can copy it down. As I scrabble through my purse to find a pen, Mom leans forward and delicately kisses the dusty computer screen, laying a wet one on her virtual lover.

— 12 —

Bring forth the best robe, and put it on him; and put a ring on his hand, and shoes on his feet.
And bring hither the fatted calf, and kill it; and let us eat, and be merry.

—Gospel according to Luke

December 23, Year Two   "Hey, Mom! Want to go to the Mall with me?"

"I need to go to the doctor, Wayne."

She has no appointment, so this is news to me. "Oh, do you? Because I was going to do some errands. But if you need to go to—"

"Oh," she says, "I don't have to go to the doctor today."

The Mall is crowded, as always, the parking lot a sea of cars. "Sears," Mom says, reading the big block letters on the building as we pull in. It's a name she recognizes; I park in another segment of the lot, ask her if she wants to come in with me.

"No," she says. "My feet hurt."

The sky is gloomy, the air cool but mild for late December. She'll be comfortable in the car.

"Foley's," she says flatly, reading again from the building we now face. "Are you going there?"

Alarms sound in my brain. No, I am not going there. It's just a store that happens to be in our line of sight at this moment. More importantly, I don't want Mom to *think* that I am going there, that she could find me there. I don't want her to think that she can find me anywhere. It's a dangerous notion, this "finding Wayne." My mission is to instill in her the belief that when I leave I am gone.

Until I return, unfindable. Non-existent. She must either come with me or stay in the car.

"No, I'm going back there," I tell her. I purposely point behind us, past the edge of her world. "It's just a big mess of stores in there," I warn. "It's a madhouse. There's so many people."

Mom agrees heartily. "I'm staying right here," she says. "I have Perry Como."

I wave goodbye, go in, do my shopping, return to the parking lot. Hmmm. Just where is the car exactly? After a few wrong turns I stumble across it. Empty. Damn. Subarus are popular here in Colorado. I've picked the wrong one. Done it before.

Still—I study the vehicle's exterior—everything about it *looks* like our car, even the idiosyncratic rust and scratch patterns etched into the primer-coated front fenders. But it isn't our car. It can't be, I reason. Mom's not in it.

I make a conscious decision to search the inside again, shading my eyes and peering through the windows like a nosy neighbor. I look on the front seat: Mom's gloves. I force the words through my brain: M-o-m-'s g-l-o-v-e-s. It's like pushing crystallized honey through a sieve. Methodically, unblinking, I scan from front seat to back to luggage area, as though I might come upon her if only I concentrate. But even this careful search fails to reveal the missing mom, and I regress to a more primitive emergency procedure: "Oh, no," I moan softly.

Four times, I remind myself accusingly. She's left the car four times. I haven't adjusted (once again) to the fact that (once again) Mom has changed. Staying in the car is not something to be depended on. That has passed. I should write it down and pin it to my sleeve.

Resigned to a wider search I turn in unsteady circles, like a tipsy Baryshnikov, scanning the field of cars. First closer in, then farther and farther out, in concentric rings until I'm on my tiptoes, hoping to catch sight of her head, a tiny grey cork bobbing in this endless ocean of metal and glass.

Flames of panic nip at me as I enter Foley's, an immediate web-work of narrow aisles and over-my-head shelving. With mounting despair I realize that I am searching not only for the proverbial needle in a haystack, but a moving needle. I can't find Mom. I can't even find my way through Foley's!

Finally, like a pinball slipping blindly past flailing flippers, I burst out into the Mall proper. I hurry down the crowded interior thoroughfare, sidestepping sluggish shoppers and scanning every face as I jog along. I pass an endless line of specialty shops, skirt the fountain, zigzag through the food court. Closing in on Sears, the other anchor store at the far end of the Mall, hope swells. That familiar name might be an anchor for Mom as well.

Sears has an airy, open feel about it. I search more efficiently, but still without success.

Out through the Sears exit, pacing the length of the building, looking out over the parking lot again from this new angle. I'm getting nowhere. Visceral alarms sound throughout my body. What makes me think she's in the Mall at all? She could have gone any direction from the car, and thanks to my useless search she's had time now to get out beyond the parking lot, across the feeder streets.

Did she head for The Salad Bowl? Would she even recognize the name from more than a year ago? I don't think so. One block west lie six lanes of constant, crazed traffic. I move off again, a hunter in search of hidden quarry, eyes and ears and cunning tuned to peak sensitivity. But with no real plan.

It's a big place. She might be here, and I might search for hours and simply never cross her path. And what if she has been kidnapped? Or injured? I've often wondered how it is that caring, loving parents lose their children. Now I know: it happens.

I check my watch. Five to three. A giddy, darkly humorous spirit settles over me. "Oh, Terry's going to be mad at me," I warn myself in hushed tones. "She gave me her mother for a couple of hours and now I've lost her!" I slip into agnostic prayer, begging a nameless Being, one which I hope is possessed of greater influence and vision than I, to "let me" find her. I continue the search, continue my whimpering mantra. "I've lost Terry's mom. I've lost Terry's mom."

Another ten minutes, another desperate visit to our still-empty car. Time to reassess. She's looking for me, I decide, or she's looking for a bathroom. Either way, she'll head for a building. Foley's was visible, and it's the one she mentioned. I charge back into the labyrinth.

I make another full circuit through the store, finishing with an inspired third lap past the perfume counter. I look to my left and, like an apparition, there she is. Upright, smiling, without visible blood or apparent injuries, clutching Perry Como with both hands.

Instant relief. All the terror and anxiety of the previous half-hour disappear, never even occurred. A dream. A nightmare.

Mom is talking to someone. A lady. And the lady has a kind but helpless look on her face. I close the distance between us quickly, never taking my eyes off of Mom, driven by the irrational but very real fear that I must get to her quickly, lest she disappear as instantaneously as she has materialized.

"Ohh," Mom exclaims happily as she catches sight of me. I throw my arm around her and she crumples into me.

The lady and I introduce ourselves. She is with Foley's Security. I wonder whether Mom went through a person or two or three to get to her, or perhaps just stumbled onto her, or she found Mom, or . . . ? These are details, like every other that takes place out of our direct experience with Mom, that I will never know.

Foley's Security releases her to my care. I thank her, and Mom and I head out together. She is excited, and breathlessly recounts the details of her adventure to Perry and to me.

"I didn't know where I was."

"What did you do?"

"I told them I was lost."

"That was good."

Her body is limp, gangly as a marionette, but the hand that grips my arm is steel.

"I was scared," she tells me.

"Me, too," I say.

Suddenly she asks, "Does anybody know?"

"No," I assure her, "just you and me."

"Well, but you're going to tell my mother."

She sounds hopeful. Sure, at least, that this is the proper thing to do. A mother has to know, after all. I am pretty certain that Terry is the mother she has in mind, pretty sure also that she will tell her about the adventure on her own.

"It's up to you," I say.

My arm around her, I pull her closer, partially supporting her, though to me she is weightless. We cuddle each other as we make our way through the crowded Mall concourse, then wade out one last time into the boundless sea. Our lifeboat awaits us.

Mom does not complain that I was gone too long. I feel no anger toward her for getting out of the car.

How could I possibly? For she was lost, and now she is found.

13

"I know where I'm going. I'm going home."

—Helen

December 24, Year Two   "Terry, I need a needle and thread," Mom tells me as we pass in the hall.

"What do you need them for?" I ask.

She doesn't answer in words, instead shows me a buttonhole on her shirt. Not a damaged buttonhole. To Mom's eye the buttonhole *is* the damage.

Christmas Day   Dinner with lots of friends and food at Jean and Dave's house. Mom enjoys herself, has a great time with the food, is ready to go as soon as the meal is finished. We persuade her to stay for some live music. She has a good time with that, too, then wants to leave as the last note dies. We mention the upcoming dessert. Mom acquiesces, loves it—and wants to leave immediately after.

On the drive home the car hums through the curves of a scenic stretch of hilly countryside.

"You couldn't pay me to live in country like this," Mom declares.

"What kind of country would you like to live in?" Wayne says.

"One with more cars."

December 27   "Wayne, look at all that snow in the driveway," Mom scolds, pointing not to the driveway I shoveled clean thirty minutes ago, but to the half-inch of snow on the concrete pad in the back yard. Theorizing that exercise and the opportunity to resolve this problem herself will do her good, I encourage her to sweep a path and offer to get her a broom. This makes her angrier. "I won't do any such thing. That's your job," she scolds, after which I hear her in her room, pleading her case to Perry Como, "Wayne doesn't do anything. It's his job."

I invite her to go on errands with me. Not interested. But a short time later I mention it again as though for the first time. "Anything to get the hell out of this house," she says.

I make my stops and we pass a pleasant hour. After lunch she invites me on a walk to look at the dogs just down the alley. We go out and she walks right up to the truck. This leads to an eerie replay of the discussion we had last summer, substituting "dogs" for "flowers." She says, "I want to go look at the dogs," and I answer, "Okay, but it's two houses down the street. We can't take a 6,000 pound truck to go fifty yards." She agrees, then says, "Let's get in the car. I want to go look at the dogs." Round and round we go.

I start laughing and hug her, albeit gingerly, because I can see that she is on the verge of falling into a sour mood again. We come to a "compromise": she will walk down the alley and I will go another way around and meet her.

When our paths cross halfway down the alley she is again in a jovial mood. We walk about eight blocks, during which time the subject of the truck, and the dogs for that matter, never comes up again. When we get home I think that she will be pleased and tired, and satisfied with our adventure. Within ten minutes, though, she is falling into a black mood and wants to go somewhere.

We continue on this seesaw—interludes of neutral or even pleasant interaction followed by Mom cursing and calling me names—through much of the day. I surprise myself by remaining emotionally level in the face of her mercurial behavior. The nastier she gets, the nicer I get. Finally she decides that she is going to go, somewhere, by herself.

"I'd rather you didn't, Mom. I'd worry about you. You might get lost."

She doesn't care. When she can't figure out how to get out either the back or front doors, she asks me to open the front.

"I don't want to open it for you, Mom. I don't think it's a good idea for you to go for a walk when you don't know where you're going."

"I know where I'm going. I'm going home."

"But your home is a thousand miles from here," I tell her. I've regressed a year, to an argument that didn't work even then.

Mom responds in kind. "My home is not that far. It's right a-round the corner."

Eventually she does get out the door. I note the time, the clothing she is wearing, which direction she is headed; I keep one eye on the clock, one eye on the streets. She returns after thirty minutes, just as I am considering a call to the police. As though law enforcement should be one's natural ally in recovering family members who have gone for a stroll.

"Glad to see you," I say. "Glad you made it back. I was worried."

She ignores me, goes to her room, tells Perry how cold she's been.

Shortly after, I leave to run a few final errands. I don't invite her, thinking she might be tired, and in any case not wanting to "reward" her reckless walking—as though she would draw any connection between the two events. That I should think she might, demonstrates only one thing: there are all kinds of thought disorders.

Supper and the rest of the evening go smoothly. Mom goes to bed, fully dressed, at 8:45.

I have learned during this day the value of expressing myself with little or no negative emotion. Say that I am worried or angry or upset? Yes. Acknowledge what I understand to be Mom's feeling? Yes. But confront, shame, or demand? No. Such responses are dangerous. Damaging. They shake the shelter of our relationship like a tornado.

December 29 This morning Mom pins her waffle to the plate with the point of her knife, then saws at it with the side of her fork.

December 30 My mother-in-law's small stash of money, with which we've been paying the rent on this house, is running low and will likely be exhausted in a few months. I decide to check into the federally funded "Section Eight" Housing assistance program in our community and learn that there is a waiting list. The anticipated time to move to the top of the list is four years.

December 31 Nine p.m. Mom's been in bed for over an hour; Wayne is in the shower; I'm seated on the closed-lid toilet, talking to him. Our one, tiny bathroom has become our prime meeting place. We use it for planning sessions and trysts. And, as now, simply visiting. It's the only room in the house with a lock.

Suddenly Mom's voice beyond the closed door: "Honey, are you in there?"

Wayne falls silent.

"Yeah, Mom. Do you need to use the bathroom?"

"Well, I could," she says with urgent nonchalance.

"Come on in." I pop up from my perch and raise the lid. "It's okay."

She sits down on the toilet, seems not to notice the sound of the water running beyond the curtain. Until Wayne makes a noise with the soap.

"What was that?" Mom asks, curious but not alarmed.

"Oh, the water's running in the shower."

Mom considers this a moment. "You going to take a shower?"

"Yeah."

We smile at each other.

"What are you going to do with that?" she asks, indicating Wayne's clothes piled in full view on the vanity top.

"I'm just going to take them out," I tell her.

Pretty soon she is up and out and a moment later I hear the "all clear" groan of her bedsprings.

Wayne likes long showers. Sometimes he sings.

Not tonight.

14

"I could walk home from here if I had a horse."

—Helen

January 2, Year Two I've been listening to my mother for an eternity, sifting her sounds from a murky early morning that covers me like a welcome blanket. That she is awake at all is uncharacteristic. But she is moving mysteriously tonight: crisscrossing her hardwood floor, roaming down the carpet-muffled hallway, her shoes clacking on the kitchen vinyl. In and out of her room, back and forth.

I pull myself from our mattress-on-the-floor bed, wondering what potion Wayne takes that he can sleep so soundly in Grand Central. The hallway is cruelly bright, flooded by the ceiling fixture that glares from beyond Mom's open door. I find her bed empty, naked. Down the hall her sheets, blankets, pillows and pillowcases are heaped like hay in front of the utility room door.

"I'm going to do laundry," Mom announces in a spritely tone.

"Mom, it's the middle of the night." I push the words out. "Let's put your sheets back on."

She considers this plan of action. "Well, I *am* tired," she concedes. Then, eyeing her bare mattress as though for the first time: "I can't sleep on a bed without sheets!"

"No."

She is very confused, unable to help. I remake the bed, get her tucked in and kissed, and go back to my own mattress, thankful that Wayne has not stripped it in my absence. Ten minutes later the alarm of Mom's squeaking springs sounds again. I check on her. She is sitting on the edge of her bed, talking contentedly to her pictures.

Two hours later she is up once more. Fully dressed, winter coat buttoned to the neck, her purse clutched in both hands.

Ready to go. Somewhere.

January 3 Mom had a good time at Cottonwood today. After her return her enthusiasm grows through the afternoon so that by 3:00 p.m. she is absolutely raving about the marvelous time she had—guys flirting with her, some kind of game or exercise at which she felt she was very proficient, a visiting dog. She wants to go back. Right now.

Five minutes ago Mom saw Wayne and me hugging, something she has surely witnessed a hundred times in the past year and a half.

"Why do you cater to Wayne so much?" she asks now, moments after he has left.

Immediately I am upset. "He's nice to you. He's nice to me," I defend.

"Well kiss my foot," she says, and goes to her room.

I don't understand why she would say such a thing. Out of curiosity as much as anything, I go to her room and ask her, careful not to burden my question with emotion or judgment, "What did you mean about me catering to Wayne so much?"

"Well," she says, "what about your husband?"

January 4 At a regular planning meeting, Terry and I meet with the Cottonwood staff. "She's a joy to be with," they tell us. "All the staff like her; some go out of their way to spend time with her." We share some of the difficulties we've been having and, on the whole, get the impression she's having a better time here than at home.

January 7 My mother is looking forward to going to Cottonwood tomorrow morning. "I have real friends," she says.

January 13 As I pull into the lot at Cottonwood just before 2 o'clock I can see my mother-in-law through the window, strained and serious-faced. By the time I switch the engine off, Wanda, a staff member, is holding the door open and Mom fairly bursts out of the doorway.

"This bitch wouldn't let me leave!" she says bitterly, striding toward the truck.

I grab at her hand as she passes me. "What are you talking about? What happened, Mom?"

Wanda joins us. Mom repeats her angry outburst and Wanda explains that Mom had a difficult hour—wanting to leave—and that she couldn't allow it because she was the only staff member present in the facility at the time. She says that Mom ripped a poster off the wall.

"I did not take a poster off!" Mom protests.

Wanda says that Mom struck her with her Perry Como picture, and called her names.

"She called *me* a bitch!" Mom counters. She doesn't want me to listen to anything Wanda has to say.

Wanda goes back into the building, returning seconds later with a crumpled drawing of some sort which she thrusts at Mom in dramatic courtroom fashion. "I didn't do that," Mom scoffs.

Wanda doesn't push it any further. "Have a good afternoon," she says to Mom. There is an edge to her tone.

Mom gets into the truck and I talk to Wanda a bit more. She explains that everything was fine until the last hour when Mom wanted to go for a walk, or perhaps to leave, to walk home, and she wasn't able to allow her to leave the building. I apologize for Mom, express my genuine concern, and suggest that we talk more at a later time. Now Wanda says that this sort of thing has happened before with others, that it's unfortunate but not serious. She will make a note that two staff need to be on duty at all times.

I join Mom in the transparent privacy of the truck. "I don't ever want to hear of you hitting people with that picture again," I tell her, shaking my forefinger for emphasis. "And if I do, I will take it away and you will never see it again!"

"Oh, ho-ho. Like hell you will," she says, full of fragile bravado.

"You just wait and see," I promise, my voice quiet, seething with control.

"Don't you wag your finger at me," she says, and again denies any name-calling of Wanda, along with whatever else she might have been accused of during my traitorous private conversation with her tormentor.

As I listen to her, I am struck by the rebellious-child role she has fallen into, as well as by the judge-and-jury persona I have taken on. She's right. I *was* wagging my finger at her. And verbally threatening her, too. I didn't realize I felt so angry. Or, until now, why.

Initially I was surprised by the whole situation, then concerned. But those feelings were soon supplanted by embarrassment and fear. I felt that I urgently needed to correct Mom, to "fix" her in order to ensure that such a thing doesn't happen again.

But, already it seems too late. What Terry and I thought was working out so well, suddenly isn't working out at all. It's falling apart, and if it continues to do so there will soon be no good day care alternative for Mom.

These thoughts tumble through my head and my heart as I sit across the tattered, torn seat from her. I am angry at her for getting into trouble, for putting these things that she does not understand—cannot understand—at risk. I am angry at her for frightening me. I am angry at her for being who she is.

Reflecting on this episode late this afternoon, I realize that I really didn't give much credence to Mom's side of the story. When Wanda said she tore a poster off the wall and Mom said "I did not," I believed Wanda. When Wanda said that Mom hit her, I believed that Mom hit her, despite Mom's denial.

Not without reason. I've seen uncountable instances in which Mom has said things that were not true, denied things that absolutely were so. In this instance she denied calling Wanda any names, although I had heard her do so only moments before. I have seen her make any kind of argument to defend herself, sometimes telling untruths, other times—perhaps unclear about the circumstance or how to express herself, perhaps with no memory of what actually happened—offering wildly improbable explanations, or simply pleading innocence. On the face of it, my bias is understandable, I think, and probably reasonably accurate.

But none of this addresses Mom's entirely natural, human need to be believed. She *has* a side. No doubt she has some feeling that she is in the right, or at least that she doesn't want to be in the wrong, as she must so often feel. However inaccurate her perception, however distorted or confused her telling, there remains the essence of a position, a perspective, that is honorable and legitimate. All she wants, after all, is to have her life.

Cottonwood can potentially offer her a place to be safe, to be fed, and to receive assistance for temporary periods when Terry and I can't be available. It can increase the odds of the three of us staying together longer. These are things I believe Mom wants, at least in the big picture. But she cannot see the big picture.

Whatever may have happened today, I feel more and more that Wanda was entirely correct in her final comment: chances of avoiding the incident would have been far better if there had been a second staff member on duty. After all, Mom simply wanted to go out the door. Maybe she wanted to find her way home and maybe that was dangerous, and maybe they have policies and liability concerns that would have overridden her request even if there had been two staff. But the core issue from Mom's perspective is that she wanted to go outside on an unarguably beautiful day (the warmest January day in Denver history, the news says this evening). How would I respond, how would *anyone* respond, in the same situation?

As day passes into evening, Mom continues off and on to bring the subject up, to describe her tortured, distorted memories of the day. "She had to make these people spit their teeth out. . . . I was there and I saw it!" she tells me, and calls Wanda vulgar names. Each time, a little bullet of fear shoots through me. But I find myself able to respond to her differently, with more compassion. I acknowledge once or twice very explicitly that I wasn't there, and that probably both of them were in the right in some respects, that each of them has a point of view.

January 14   "I could walk home from here if I had a horse," my mother-in-law suddenly tells me as I finish up a few breakfast dishes on this Sunday morning.

"Where would home be, Mom? Where would you tell the horse to go?"

"I don't know. . . ." She looks forlorn, tired. "I guess I shouldn't have ever come down here," she says.

"Why?"

"Because I don't know how to get back."

January 20   "Terry, I had the worst day of my life," Mom told me today when I picked her up at Cottonwood. It's hard to ignore such statements.

On the other hand, after dinner this evening when Wayne says, "Terry and I don't clean our plates as well as you do, Mom," she replies, "Neither does Ella. That's because she has her lights on."

That is easier to ignore.

January 22   My mother-in-law is having some confusion about edible and inedible. It seems bizarre that she can't tell the nut from the shell. And yet, I can see how it's akin to my sometimes forgetting why I came into a room, or making a mental note of two things I want to tell Terry, and within seconds being able to remember only one.

I take for granted that I can discriminate food from non-food, but my ability to do so is a learned one. If I were to lose, even for a moment, my memory of the distinction between shell and nut, then why would I *not* chew one as likely as the other?

January 23   I ask Terry's mother to sign some insurance and medical release documents. She does so without hesitation. "They won't put me in jail, will they?" she jokes, but doesn't read the papers or ask anything about them. She has not in the longest time asked about anything having to do with her financial matters. She never has money in her purse, often makes that observation, but seems not in the least disturbed by the fact. I think that she no longer has any notion that she owns a mobile home or that there are bills being paid on it, or that I have been tending to her financial affairs for almost a year and a half.

This is another loss, but a kind of pleasant one. In the most unexpected of ways Mom has attained financial independence.

February 1   My mother is getting slower and slower starts to Cottonwood. Today she refuses to go altogether.

February 7   Difficulties accumulate at Cottonwood. The most prevalent: Mom wants to continue on walks when staff want her to return to the facility so that they can be available to meet other clients' needs. Terry and I have also received reports of her striking staff. Two days ago they called and asked that we pick her up early.

They describe her behavior as "combative." I find this to be not only an ugly term—one which conjures up an image of someone raging out of control, aggressively seeking out victims, fond of fighting—but an unfair and inaccurate one as well. Like all labels, it suggests that the quality in question is an intrinsic and defining one. No allowance is made for circumstance. Mightn't it be more accurate to say of my mother-in-law that *sometimes* she is combative *here at Cottonwood*? Or, better yet, that *sometimes we staff here at Cottonwood find ourselves in conflict with Helen*?

Without a doubt, Cottonwood does not have the resources—the funding, ultimately—to meet every need of every one of its clients. But neither does Mom have the resources to understand why she should end her unfinished walk at the request of someone she does not know, or why she should not physically resist when her verbal refusal proves ineffective.

Is she combative, or merely a woman taking a stroll? Is it her shortcoming, or Cottonwood's, or that of a society which does not fully provide for the legitimate needs of its weaker members?

February 9   An Adult Protective Services caseworker from the Department of Social Services appears at our door. Her name is Tammy and I've never met her before. She says that she "just wants to know how things are going with Helen at day care" and, in general, how our lives are going. I invite her in.

"I was at Cottonwood yesterday, observing," she tells me, and seems to be aware of some of the difficult situations that have arisen between the staff and my mother-in-law. "Are there other services that she needs?" she wonders.

Terry's and my business, and along with it our personal economy, have been at a near standstill for eighteen months. Financial compensation for the care we provide to Mom would lighten that burden, might make it possible to continue doing what we are doing for a significantly longer period of time and to do it with less stress and distraction. Does this fall into the category of "other services that she needs"? It does in my book.

But when I move to take advantage of Tammy's serendipitous offer by raising the compensation question she replies, "No, we don't pay families for providing care." They pay Cottonwood to provide respite care, she reminds me. They'll pay for a few hours per week of in-home assistance provided by a professional agency. They'll pay for services provided by a nursing home.

I point out that my mother-in-law is not well suited to facility settings, partly because of her frequent desire to leave whatever place she's in at the moment. "As for home health services," I tell her, "even if it were a benefit to her or to us, I can't imagine that she would tolerate the presence of a stranger in the house. She wouldn't understand what it's all about. And isn't family care a better solution anyway?" I ask. "That way she could remain in an environment that's familiar, and be cared for by people she knows."

As though it were an actual response to what I have said, Tammy says again that they don't provide that.

Tammy strikes me as an amiable person. She is well-informed and clear-spoken, and I have no doubt that what she says is accurate. But I am searching for something more than accuracy, some passion in her voice, some fire in her soul that reaches beyond the margins of the *status quo*. She may not have the authority to provide the solutions I desire, but can she imagine them? Does she have an opinion about them? Does she have a better way?

Tammy says that money is a basic issue. They can't afford to pay a home-care worker $14/hour, 24 hours per day, 30 days a month. It's more economical to pay a nursing home the $2,400 or so after the client's Social Security contribution.

"I understand that money is a limiting factor," I tell her, "and I accept that. But why not provide that same $2,400—or maybe even just the seven or eight hundred you pay to Cottonwood—directly to the family and allow *them* to take care of the person in their own home? Especially for clients like my mother-in-law, who don't need nursing care."

"That's not what we do," she says.

Serendipity is a fleeting thing.

15

Split the stick, you find me there;
lift the stone, there am I.

—Gnostic Gospel of St. Thomas

February 21, Year Two   Mom woke us this morning at
4 a.m., banging around the house and telling people to "be quiet,
because Terry and Wayne are sleeping." Today she seems more alert
and energetic than ever. Unlike ourselves.

We've been talking, Terry and I, about Mom's need and our
desire for community. Our resources are simply not sufficient:
money is running out, we have a desperately needed work trip
scheduled in April, Mom's brain power is diminishing. There have
been several incidents at Cottonwood recently, two of them resulting in calls to pick Mom up early, and the staff has suggested medication to modify her behavior.

For eighteen months we have been trying to find ways to reverse, halt, or slow the progress of this disease. In addition to the
conventional medical care provided by Mom's doctor, we've taken
her to a wide array of alternative healthcare professionals, consulted
with M.D.s by telephone, filled her with vitamins and minerals and
any supplement that suggests the slightest possibility of relief. We
have not succeeded, which is to say, not in any dramatic, irrefutable,
or all-encompassing way. The thing that seemed most helpful last
fall was an increase in thyroid medication recommended by an out-
of-state physician with whom we consulted. Mom's primary doctor
went along with it for awhile, but by mid-December, when blood
tests suggested her thyroid levels were high, the doctor was adamant
about backing off. Each decrease in thyroid dosage since that time

has seemed to be followed by a decrease in Mom's abilities about a week later. Her confusion is deepening, and her overall function during the past couple of weeks has diminished in every sphere.

I know that there are individuals who do caregiving for years—as long as needed—with little or no relief, but I don't know if Terry and I can count ourselves among them. I don't know that we have the emotional or physical strength, the financial capability, the generosity. We want help, need help, help which makes Mom more able. Or failing that, help which provides us with enough assistance to meet her needs, and ours. We have talked all these issues over with her doctor, who has prescribed a tranquilizer, oxazepam, for acute episodes of anger or agitation, as well as an antidepressant, sertraline. My gut feeling is that mood- and behavior-altering drugs are the wrong way to go, that they will merely address symptoms, whereas we want to address causes. We feel virtually certain, for instance, that Mom is not depressed. She has many moods, a good appetite and energy level, and exhibits a very definite interest in life. Her problem, and ours, is how to make her life work. I fear that these medications will not accomplish that, might even diminish her abilities or life experience in the bargain. In agreeing to their use do we not make ourselves co-conspirators, allowing society to avoid for yet one more day the responsibility of finding better, more fully humane answers to the problem at hand?

Our dilemma is one faced by millions: difficult behaviors displayed over a prolonged period, even if they are "merely" symptoms, can be exhausting for all involved. Terry and I have sought help, but we have sought it from a doctor. And while the doctor may wish for it as much as we, she cannot write a prescription for a better society. There are no other choices in sight. We have agreed to give the medications a try.

March 4 Mom seemed somewhat calmer for about a week after starting the new meds. Since then we have seen little or no benefit. If anything, it seems she's been more angry and upset, not happy with anything. And there are the unwanted effects. Wayne and I have both seen hand tremors. She's had sleep disturbances and paranoia. And she's been wetting herself, reminding us that urinary incontinence was chronic when she was on so many medications for years prior to living with us. Listed side effects of the medications she is currently taking include urinary frequency, urgency, and incontinence, as well as confusion, agitation, headache, tremors, depression, and paranoia.

If the drugs would work, fine. We can't see much evidence of that. They make her dopey and unhealthy—not even happy. This evening, during a period of tremors and Mom's complaint of headache, we wonder if she is having a stroke.

About three weeks ago, it became apparent to us that Mom had found time to strike up something of a relationship with one of the few older male clients at Cottonwood. We'd seen William a few times. He's a stand-out-in-the-parking-lot, when's-my-ride-going-to-get-here? kind of guy—probably how he and Mom met!—a tall, wiry fellow about Mom's age who speaks little and seems to cast a wary, perceptive eye on everything about him. Mom calls him "the old man."

She came home from Cottonwood one day in mid-February with an unusual complaint:

Mom: They took all the feeling away.
Wayne: They took all your feelings away?
M: Yep.
Terry: How'd they do that?
M: You just don't have any more feelings.
W: Is that good? . . . Or bad?
M: No, bad.
W: How did you know that they were gone? What did it feel like?
M: I just . . . (open hand to chest) feel it in here.
T: So you didn't have any feelings left?
M: The old man was giving me all my feelings. (laughs) All the clouds were coming in and I thought, we're not going to go any-

where with these black clouds. So that's when we decided, me and the old man.

T: Mmhmm. What'd you decide?

M: We decided we weren't going to come.

W: Seems like a pretty smart fellow. Got a lot of common sense.

M: He says to me, he says, "The skies are getting real dark." He says, "Don't you go driving out there. The skies are too dark for you."

T: I like this guy. He looks out for you.

Today William and his son arrived at Cottonwood at the same time as we. Wayne and I introduced ourselves to the son, Todd. "My mother really likes your dad," I said. "They seem to be friends."

He nodded. "This place is good for us," he said, "but not so good for them."

After Mom and William went in, I told Todd that Wayne and I are thinking about having William over to our house. He liked the idea. "Saturday or Sunday," I said, "which would be better?" He didn't think it would matter.

My spirits rose, and by the time we got home we were fantasizing romance and marriage and happily ever after; putting together scenarios of our two families sharing the care of our two parents. A new twist on blended families. An idea that even then we realized was barely one-tenth-baked.

This evening, watching Mom's hand tremble like an aspen leaf in a September breeze, everything seems different. Everything is unraveling. She could be dead tomorrow. I have this thought: if she would die in her sleep, it would be a good thing.

March 5   Worries are piling up, little things and big. My mother's incontinence is creating lots of extra laundry, the washer isn't working right, no dryer, and I just hung the clothes out and now it looks like rain. We're so far down that even a clouded sky spells disaster to us. Money is running out, much work remains yet to prepare for a month-long business trip in April, and the situation with Mom's mobile home—we stopped paying the lot rent two months ago—is coming to a head.

Tonight Mom and I sing "Pennies From Heaven" and it's a feat for me to keep up with her many new lyrics. She's very happy, joking, doing really well. Twenty-four hours ago we thought she might be dying.

March 9 William's circumstance has changed. His family is putting him into respite care, perhaps leading to a nursing home placement.

Without warning we received a letter from Cottonwood this week saying they won't accept my mother-in-law more than half-days, effective immediately. We had to cancel a one-day out of town trip. Yesterday I talked with Mom's current caseworker at Social Services and expressed a lot of anger about the restrictions on funding for home care assistance. I was still angry this morning, taking it out on Terry especially, sometimes in front of Mom. Name-calling, bitching, moaning.

This afternoon I'm at Mass with Mom, our usual Saturday custom. When I parked at the curb she wanted to know, "What the hell are we stopping here for?" It's a question she's asked nearly every week for eighteen months, unconvinced when I tell her "church" until we step inside the doors.

In the opening song we ask God for forgiveness for our shortcomings and misdeeds. We're singing this song, which is to say, *I'm* singing. Mom's book is open to some random page, her hand tracking across the paper as though following the verse, her lips mouthing voiceless words. As we return to the refrain, I privately direct my request for forgiveness to Mom. I am keenly aware that I was harsh and negative with her today. So I sing the line, turning my head toward her with that thought in my mind.

Just that quickly I have a notion, an actual sensation would be more accurate, that it isn't Mom standing next to me at all, but God. That this elderly, demented woman, who can't find her page, who sometimes doesn't hold the book right side up, is God herself.

She is God in disguise, as in the old tale in which God appears as a beggar at the door to see how she will be received. I am shaken, figuratively and literally. A shudder rushes through me and tears well in my eyes.

A dozen years ago, snorkeling for the first time off a Kauai beach, I dipped my head below the surface and was astounded to find myself immersed in a universe of color and form and living creatures that I had neither seen nor imagined to exist before that instant.

I feel now as I felt then, only more so. Blind, but now I see.

March 10   Wayne's dream:

> *Terry and Mom and I are in the car. I am driving along a winding mountain road. Suddenly we're in a turn, sliding on ball bearing gravel. I fight the skid, fight the panic, but there comes a moment when I have the awful realization that I can't hold it, that we are going over the edge.*
>
> *We burst through the papier-mâché guardrail, cut a path through shrubs and rock toward free fall. I am terrified, and tormented by guilt for taking Terry and Mom with me. I let go of the wheel, grab each of them by the hand. "I'm sorry," I say as we plummet. We are all scared. Falling.*
>
> *It is a nightmare plunge that goes on and on. I find time to recall the old Bible story of Satan tempting Jesus to cast himself off the cliff, and I begin to pray to God to send his angels to us. But I can't do it. In dreams it seems, even as in waking life, I find it difficult to pray to the God I was raised on. I speak instead to the angels directly: "Save us!" I implore. "Catch the car and ease it down to a safe landing."*
>
> *It seems preposterous, even in my dream, but I have a hope: our little Subaru gliding to a feather landing, just as I myself have done in so many flying dreams in the past.*
>
> *The prayers and images come and go, and still we fall. And fall. And continue to fall. Weightless, waiting for the annihilating impact.*
>
> *Suddenly we are driving along again, but now on a road far below. Mom and Terry seem to have no memory of the near crash, no sense that anything out of the ordinary has occurred.*

But I do. I am certain, in fact, that we have been saved. Not by God, or luck, or Subaru engineering. By angels.

March 11 My mother and I are in the bathroom, a place that as often as not serves as her dressing room these days. I've already selected her outfit. The job we struggle with now is getting the simple garments *on* her. Even with my help, dressing has become a formidable task for Mom, doubly hobbled as she is by the limitations of an aging, wounded body, and a mind that is more easily fooled now by this puzzle called clothes.

And to make matters worse, today she is distracted. With one arm through a sleeve she stops, looks at me.

"No, that was it, Mom. You had it."

I gently guide the other sleeve over her other hand and arm. Again she pauses, studies me some more. Hands over head, the blouse shimmies down and Mom's head pops out, all smiles at this success. Again she surveys me, top to bottom.

"I keep lookin' at ya," she says, "to see what you're made of."

"What do you think?"

"Sugar and spice and everything nice."

March 12 Mom spots the laundry Terry hung out just an hour ago. For some time now laundry flapping in a breeze has bothered her, and today is no exception. She wants to take it down, to fold it, to organize and neaten life. I do my best to discourage her with explanations and distractions, but she is persistent. "Couldn't I just give it a try?" she implores.

It's a request I find hard to resist. "Okay," I relent with a smile, "give it a try."

She returns, her basket brimming with neatly folded clothes. "I only brought in the dry things," she says happily.

And she is almost right.

March 17 Hardly back in the house after our third excursion of the day, my mother says she wants to go for a walk. I refuse, and she's out the door in a huff. With a sigh of resignation, I note the time: 2:55.

An hour later Wayne and I are once again taking turns driving around town and listening for the phone. It's my turn in the car. I am a public menace, racing everywhere, from downtown to the city limits and back again. The car drives itself; my eyes search everywhere at once. I look in the church, the grocery, all her favorite haunts. Dark and cold press ever closer.

At 5 p.m. my heart hammers equally with embarrassment and fear as Wayne calls the police. Before he can finish his explanation, though, the dispatcher tells him that they have just picked up someone answering Mom's description.

The location is far beyond the bounds of our search. She made it to, and somehow crossed, six lanes of federal highway, proceeded north another mile, and then went into an auto parts store. A clerk there, recognizing her impairment, called the police and an officer picked her up and brought her to the station. An identification tag on her purse went for naught. The police officer noticed and asked about the telephone number on it, but took Mom at her word when she said it wasn't her number.

A police vehicle pulls up to our curb. I can see Mom in the back, behind the wire-mesh screen. The female officer, her hips bedecked with gun, baton, flashlight, cuffs and more, gently assists Mom from the vehicle. Wayne and I, unsure of the proper protocol, wait at the door, drenched in relief. Mom and the officer are halfway up the walk when Mom abruptly stops. Beaming, she spreads her arms wide and announces with joyful pride: "I'm in jail!"

April 6 "Forty-nine years ago, on Easter Sunday morning, you were in the hospital having me," I tell Mom as soon as she rises this morning.

"Really?"

"Really."

"I'll be damned."

I tell her the story of the delivery—Dr. Frank rooting for a boy with cheers of, "Come on, Russell Joseph," his nurse urging, "Come on, Terry Marie." I recount my sunrise birth, the cord around my neck, the caul that covered my face. It is a story that she has told me countless times over the years.

Today, for Mom, it is a new story altogether.

April 8   The doctor recently discontinued Mom's sertraline and oxazepam. Buspirone and clorazepate—both anti-anxiety agents— have been added.

April 9   Skimming down the highway toward the airport to deposit Terry's mother on her flight to Sharon's house in California and ourselves on the road to Kansas and the start of our big spring tour, it seems like there is plenty of time. But that's before the trickster EGR light suddenly bathes the instrument panel in red. That's before we stand in the wrong check-in line until our legs are crumpling beneath us. That's before we misjudge the time Mom needs to make the long journey from window to gate. Such things take their toll. Which is how I come now to find myself sprinting the final yards to that very gate, arriving just in time to watch through the window as the door to the plane slams shut.

I explain Mom's situation in breathless, urgent tones to the lady at the counter, all the while pointing to Terry and her mom, now only yards away, gliding toward us on the automated walkway. I am a tad excited and wild in the eye I'm sure, but there the plane sits, and here we are, and I fully expect that they will re-open the door and let this little old demented lady on board. The airline employee efficiently disabuses me of this notion and, as if the behemoth beyond the glass is activated by her words, the plane—Mom-less— separates from the entry tunnel and begins to roll slowly, surreally, away.

"We waited in line a long time," I tell the lady at the counter. "We hurried down here as fast as we could go. The ticket counter person said she would call about us."

The plane recedes.

I must stop it, reverse its motion, reverse time itself if necessary. By turns I insist, cajole, demand, raise my voice, hurl vulgarities and, finally, as the plane taxis toward the runway, spew inflammatory mutterings on the topic of understanding now why one should always bring a gun to the airport.

Several airline personnel take notice. They gather now in a wary knot behind the check-in counter. One threatens to summon Security, and I retain just enough sense of self-preservation to dampen my display. Or perhaps it is that I can do little else, for at this moment, when Security is just a button-push away, I am brought unexpectedly to a halt by my own physiology.

My heart throbs in my chest; my tongue has grown to twice its size and wears a cotton sock; my diaphragm is in spasm. I can't pull in air. I can't speak or breathe. I have never felt these sensations in my life.

The plane—the once all-important plane—has departed the gate, and my mind as well. Travel dilemmas, even the possibility of arrest, have receded to a distant corner of my brain. I hear nothing but the pounding engine and screeching valves inside my own body. I am thinking heart attack. Stroke. Death.

I do not speak or move. I don't know for how long.

"You don't need to call Security," I assure the staring group hunched behind the bulwark counter when a measure of sanity and physiological equilibrium return.

Shaken by my brush with death, listing heavily under a burden of shame and embarrassment, I break my siege and approach Terry and Mom, who have taken refuge a short distance away. I can see the fury at me in Terry's face, but she holds herself in check. I look to my mother-in-law, fearing the worst, that my outburst has unhinged her. But I see at once that she is possessed of herself, on a far more even keel than I. Although not entirely at ease, perceiving perhaps only the essence of the past few minutes—that something has gone badly for her family—she has weathered the storm the best of all of us. She turns to Terry. "Help him," she gently urges.

Three restless hours later Mom boards a flight to San Diego, appearing none the worse for wear. Exhausted and several hours behind schedule, Terry and I head eastward on the first leg of the most extensive school trip we have ever scheduled.

Alone together in the car, Denver International Airport's "Rocky Mountain" roof line receding in the rearview mirror, Terry speaks her mind. She tells me that my behavior has caused her immense pain, reminds me that instead of rolling toward the land of Dorothy and Toto I could be sitting at this moment in a cell, our hard-earned trip scuttled, our career in tatters, and our future—as a family, as a couple, as individuals—in jeopardy.

Other than to murmur agreement and a meek "I'm sorry," I do not speak. Silently, I thank whatever gods there may be for good luck, and for a wife far better.

April 10   Wayne and I have treated ourselves to a Bed & Breakfast, a beautiful and intriguing place, perched like a castle on the wide plains of eastern Colorado. . . .

I wake in the middle of the night and wander the hall outside our second floor room, look down into the large entry parlor, sit in a comfy chair and listen to piped-in music of the '50s and '60s. I start to smile, something I haven't done in a long time. . . .

This morning I am greeted by the sun rising over the prairie. Lovely. And at breakfast—a cornucopia of fresh fruits, pastries, eggs, meats, and juices—I spy a Lewis Carroll quote on a twenty-foot banner over the dining room windows: "Why, I have sometimes believed as many as six impossible things before breakfast!"

Everything about this place cheers me. I'm feeling happy, looking forward to our visit at the local school.

Anything is possible.

April 12   When the phone rings in our room at the conference hotel in St. Louis, it startles us. It's Sharon, calling to tell Terry and me that Mom was thrown out of the day care program they had arranged. It was her first day. The reasons for her dismissal are not entirely clear to me. Walking out? Shouting? Being combative? Who knows.

April 19 We completed the eighth school visit of our trip today and have had numerous contacts through the week with Sharon and Denny.

Two days ago they told us that Terry's mother did not get on well at a new day care, where she was put in a room to eat by herself and somehow got outside. When the staff came after her she threw pebbles and sticks at them. The police were summoned. National emergency.

A friend of Terry's here in St. Louis, an experienced geriatrics nurse, suggested a temporary hospital placement. "She's miserable," she told us. "She can't come home right away, so why not try something different?" Sharon and Denny were miserable; Mom was miserable. It seemed like it might be some sort of temporary solution, giving Sharon and Denny a break and Mom, too, while providing an evaluation of her medications.

Yesterday they called to fill us in. Mom has been admitted to a general psychiatric ward at a local hospital. She has been placed on new medication, including risperidone, an antipsychotic. She is incontinent of bladder and bowel. The staff there have raised the possibility that they will seek a temporary, possibly permanent, non-family conservatorship—some sort of guardianship, we presume—for Mom.

Everything is being taken out of our hands. Literally overnight, we have lost all practical input into decisions being made, the effects of which could be long lasting. Permanent.

"I can't believe it," Terry tells me through her tears. "I just wanted everyone to have a break. I wanted her medications evaluated. I didn't want her stuck in some place for 72 hours and drugged! Letting her urinate all over herself. That wasn't the point! The point was to figure out what she needs, and to provide it."

April 20 We call the hospital. She sounds heavily tranquilized, and can't get my name. "Torry?" she tries. Despite this worrisome start, the conversation is almost pleasant. She clearly knows who Wayne and I are. Once, when she and I begin speaking at the same time, Mom recognizes this. "Go ahead," she says. "Perry Como's still with me," she wants us to know. "Come and see me." It's so good to talk to her again.

For two days we have been sending her love and prayers, uniting our spirits with hers. It makes us feel better. Her, too, we hope.

April 22 We departed St. Louis and arrived in Hays, Kansas yesterday evening. Today we make calls to Mom's Colorado doctor and the social worker connected with her office. Neither is in. Their return calls end up on our Voice Mail in Colorado.

Sharon says that Mom's doctor at the hospital doesn't want our input, or theirs. If we want to talk to him we will have to make an appointment. Sharon has found that there is an Alzheimer's unit at a nearby hospital, but no transfer seems to be in the works. Meanwhile Mom is urinating on herself, smearing feces on the walls, and not eating well. How can she? Sharon says that they gave her two spoons with which to eat chicken fried steak.

April 23 Our last school on this first portion of our spring tour: Colby, Kansas. The librarian is totally organized. The kids and teachers are prepared, calm, involved. Our host feeds us lunch, complete with homemade dessert. We give thanks.

April 24 Back home for a few days before next week's school engagements on the Western Slope. Sharon says that Mom is still at the same hospital. Her stay has been extended fourteen days. There will be no transfer to the Alzheimer's unit, this, at least in part, because the doctor in charge of her treatment believes that she is not mentally competent to sign herself into that presumably more appropriate setting. Apparently this was less of an issue when she arrived at his hospital. As Terry and I understand it, the doctor's main concern is that his patient is talking to a picture of Perry Como.

* * * * *

"Hello, Mom? . . . Hi, Mom! This is Terry. . . Somebody's yelling at your ear? Are you okay? . . . Are you okay? . . . You think you're getting better? That's good. How are you feeling? . . . About the same? . . . Lots of people are standing around, huh? . . . It'll be a while till what? . . . It'll be a while till you come home? Well, I sure hope you feel better and better . . . It is getting better? I'm so glad! . . . How's the food there? . . . The food is fine? . . . Good. How are you sleeping? . . . What did you say, Mom? Talk a little louder . . . Can you put your mouth closer to the telephone? . . . Oh, good, yes you are. You're talking right into the telephone. . . . You'd like to find a better place to stay? Is that what you said? . . . What? . . . Say that again. . . . Oh, I wish I could come over there. I'm so far away right now, though. I can't come over right now or I would. . . . Yeah, I'm a thousand miles away. So that's why I'm not over there. . . . What, Mom? What are you gonna do? Well, you just get better. . . . What? . . . Yeah, let's hope it gets better. . . . You know what? We're thinking about you and we love you. . . . Okay. Good. . . . What was that last part? I couldn't hear you. You want to what? . . . Oh, you'd like to . . . Where would you like to come? . . . You'd like to come over here? . . . But you don't know how to get here. . . . Yeah. We'll work on that, Mom. And we love you. . . . What? . . . Bring Wayne along? I will."

April 29 Terry's mother will be released from the hospital to come back to us on May 4, the day we return from the final leg of our tour. Based on what we have heard from Sharon and Denny and from Mom herself in our phone conversations, and knowing that she has been heavily medicated for weeks, we believe that she will need special care when she returns.

After visiting several nursing homes that have special Alzheimer's units we have made arrangements through Mom's doctor to have her admitted to Holly Hills Health Care for a 30-day stay. A trial period for permanent placement if everything goes well, or a respite for all of us while she gets through her medication withdrawal.

Today we go back on the road for our final week of school visits.

16

"I want to live here."

—Helen

May 4, Year Two   When my mother gets off the plane she looks about as bad as I could have imagined. Her hair is plastered flat against pasty skin from the top of her forehead to the nape of her neck. She is walking, with Sharon's help, but her body looks at once both familiar and unfamiliar to me, as though Sharon lugs beside her a life-sized but inaccurate doll replica of our mother. Her arms are slack at her side, her legs rubbery and her posture sagging and rounded as though her skeleton and muscles cannot hold her. Somehow she shuffles the length of the corridor from the plane to the gate where Wayne and I wait. She has aged twenty years in the 25 days since we last saw her. I have never seen such a transfiguration.

Several times during our journey through the crowded concourse she starts to remove her blouse. "So I can go to bed," she explains weakly.

May 5   The sermon drones on. My eyes have fallen shut, searching for the rest they could not find last night. I feel myself weaving, catch myself, open my eyes, see Terry's mother weaving next to me. A matched set.

She stopped participating in the Sign of Peace greeting months ago, but today a little boy with dark hair and darker eyes reaches far across the pew toward her, as though to reach her is his special mission. Mom is oblivious to him, but he does not relent. He holds his arm out until it wavers of its own weight, stretches himself another inch closer. Suddenly she sees him, grasps his hand, and shakes it long and warmly. Although I've just witnessed it, she tells me now about the incident with great pride, her loving eye still on the boy.

A short-haired woman stands directly in front of Mom. Two feet away. Mom gives me a stage whisper, with which I have learned to live over the many months she's been using them. "This man in front here has earrings," she informs me and a sizeable portion of the congregation. "I don't go for that."

She doesn't want to go to communion, tells me so two or three times as the Mass progresses. When the time comes and I rise to go, I am torn. But for an occasional good hymn, communion is the heart of the ceremony for me, the only thing I find energy in. But I am afraid today to leave her here alone.

"Do you want to go to communion?" I ask nonchalantly, one more time.

"Sure," she says.

She walks slowly, feeling her way with her feet, although the floor is flat and smooth, grasping each pew as she passes. Instinctively, I move out into the center of the wide aisle and walk beside rather than behind her. She takes my hand. We walk at her speed, much slower than the communicants ahead, and a gap quickly opens in front of us, broadening with every passing second.

It appears that the communion-givers serving our line will soon be temporarily unemployed. But before disaster can strike, communicants from the other line stream across the aisle in front of us, filling the gap like rush hour drivers finding a lucky lane change opportunity on a congested urban highway. Just as quickly, their places are taken by those behind them, as well as by other aisle-crossers who have been languishing behind Mom and me. It must be a thing of beauty for those in the choir loft above. Catholics are nothing if not proficient in church-related traffic maneuvers.

Although there are two communion servers for our line, when we reach the front we improvise again and approach one of them together, still holding hands. That's the key, I realize as the wafer is presented. That's what got us here, our own private communion.

After Mass we burst into the light of secular day and cross the street for a quick visit to the supermarket. Mom shows a surprising recollection of the premises. She knows where the bathrooms are located, where Paul Newman resides, and where they keep the candy bars. Although since her return yesterday she has struggled to find, or identify when shown, our dining table at home, she seems to know pretty much everything one needs to know about a modern supermarket.

After lunch I offer her a walk in our neighborhood and she leads me straight across the street, toward the yard with the beautiful flowering crab that she's been admiring since her return. She can't remember what it's called, although we've named it for her every time she asks. Mostly she refers to it as "that tomato bush," despite the fact that it is a large, mature tree, 25 feet tall and just as broad. Her love for this tree is without limit and, as we walk hand in hand along the fence, her fervor hatches a plan.

"Let's see if they wanna sell it," she urges, entirely serious. I think she would like to have it forever.

"Well," I begin thoughtfully, as though her suggestion teeters just on the edge of possibility, "it's a pretty big tree. It'd be pretty hard."

Mom considers this a moment. "Well," she suggests, "if they say no, we'll just tell them, 'We were just asking.' "

A few steps further on, suddenly conscious of our hand-holding, Mom whispers conspiratorially in my ear, "We don't have to tell anybody we're not married." It seems a prudent strategy. We go right on along, all the way around the block, and whether we are friends, young lovers, or aging in-laws, no one along our route is the wiser.

On our way up the alley we come across a family working in their yard. Mom quickly notes that they, too, have a crab apple tree. Soon the family dog comes to bark at us through the fence, in a friendly but tree-guarding fashion, and then the young man comes over to greet us. Mom and he introduce themselves. His name is

Bob. They shake hands, Bob first removing his work glove in chival-rous fashion.

"This is my son-in-law Wayne," she tells Bob, and I feel suddenly pleased, lucky somehow, to be standing beside her. She tugs on my sleeve. I follow her gaze, beyond Bob, beyond Bob's dog, beyond Bob's much-prized crab apple tree, to where Mrs. Bob, presumably, and a towheaded toddler are setting tiny, two-leafed plants in fresh, friable earth.

"Would you like to sell some of those strawberries?" Mom asks Bob.

"Of course, they don't have any yet," I say, hoping with seven words to explain about strawberries to Mom and about Mom to Bob.

"You can have all you want," Bob says, as though the harvest were imminent. "Any that we don't take into the kitchen."

Bob doesn't need any explanations.

May 6 This morning, both my mother-in-law's doctor and the nurse were excited about how much better Mom looks than they expected.

Everybody's been telling us for months and months and months, doctors and social workers in particular, that we have to take care of ourselves, from which I inferred that they thought that we were not. So how is it that today—hardly more than a week after the doctor and we agreed on a nursing home admission and on the very day she is expected to be admitted, a day when Terry and I are more physically, mentally, and emotionally exhausted than ever, a day when Mom is not even 48 hours beyond the worst shape I've ever seen her in—how is it that today everybody is saying she looks good? How is it that we're having to shake our heads and say, "It's not what it appears—she's *not* doing well"?

Yes, she does look good. But that's only because Terry has washed and set her hair. Because she's bathed her, fed her, and provided love and affection to overflowing. Because we've provided the salves of music, and flowers, and fresh air. Because for forty-eight hours we've given her constant attention. She looks good, and she still has a lot of social skills—that's part of what the doctor and nurse were seeing—but she's not *doing* well.

Her sleep pattern, which was always so good, has been disturbed these past two nights. She was animated to the point of agitation both evenings, getting to bed late and sleeping intermittently. Last night she spent two hours fumbling with the locks on the front door. I feigned sleep on the couch, watching through slitted eyes the entire time. Mom was not fooled, and repeatedly pleaded, sometimes demanded, that I help her. I was touched by the poignancy of her dilemma—trying so hard, applying every skill she had, but just unable to manage two locks and a chain. Part of me wanted to go and help her, to take a midnight stroll together. Maybe that was all that would have been needed. . . .

Finally, she gave up. "Mom, you're tired," I told her. "Let's go to bed." I led her more than once to her room, but she would not enter, as though it had become a tainted, unsafe place. She doesn't seem to really own it as hers like she did before, even after her returns from previous trips. She recognized it then, and was glad to be back. Now, she doesn't seem to have any real recognition of this home we share.

When she became wholly exhausted, sometime after midnight, she lay down in the living room, on the floor, and dozed instantly.

She's been incontinent since her return, two or three times each night. She's tried to get up, sometimes found the bathroom and sometimes not, but in each case long past the time when she needed it. And once in the bathroom, day or night, she doesn't seem to know very well anymore what a toilet is or how to use it.

Question: What do you do with toilet paper after you've used it?

a.   put it in the waste can
b.   throw it on the floor
c.   tuck it neatly into the center of the current toilet paper tube
d.   wipe the lavatory bowl and counter top with it

Although it was never a tough question for her before, during the past two days Mom has chosen

e.   all of the above

Her conversation is not as sensible as it was a month ago. Terry and I have always been good at reading between the lines and learning her new language as it has evolved, but it seems to have taken a quantum leap in the past twenty-six days. Yesterday, at lunch:

"I was going to go home today" Mom tells Terry as she washes vegetables for the lunch salad. "I was going to build myself a castle."
"You were?"
Her mother laughs. "Yeah."
"What were you going to build it out of?"
"Well, you know, just out of different things. I said, 'I can do that.'" She hesitates, then continues with another small laugh. "I don't think I really can, but . . . I was gonna do it. . . . I have already built things. And got a good reference for it."
"Have you? Like what?"
"Well, things that needed this and needed that and, uh, things that were missing things."
"Mmhmm."
"I did. But I don't remember how I did it anymore. . . . I could probably build something somewhere else one of these days, and wouldn't even know what it's about."

For all these reasons, Terry and I have reaffirmed our decision of a week ago that if ever we are going to explore nursing home placement—and it seems we must before very long—this is the time to do it. This time when Mom is so physically compromised, so confused, showing so little recognition of and taking so little solace in the home we have shared for nearly two years.

We talked with her this morning about the possibility of her living in a different place. She responded positively, seemed to find it an agreeable idea.

The admitting nurse from Holly Hills comes to the house this afternoon and talks to Mom and us about her moving there today. Mom smiles, though weakly, and agrees again.

We are alone now. Mom sits with Terry and me on the couch, the three of us in a line, not looking at one another. "I want to live *here*," she says quietly. Words that tear our hearts.

* * * * *

"I'm driving," I tell Wayne when we meet at the car. I dig for my keys, stop, look up at him. "I should drive," I say again. He steps aside, goes around and slips into my usual place in the seat behind my mother.

For the first few blocks there is an unnatural silence in the car, but Mom soon breaks it by reading signs along the roadside. The anxiety she expressed only minutes ago about moving has disappeared altogether. Our destination appears to be as far from her awareness as it is close to mine.

"I'm happy that you're going to be so close, Mom," I say.

"Oh, yeah," Wayne agrees. "I was so upset when you were in California, Mom. You were too far away then. This is going to be much better."

"Look at these flowers," she says, pointing out the window. . . . "Looks like it's gonna rain. . . . Look at these flowers."

I stop at the light. "No turn on red," she reads.

We arrive at Holly Hills. I pull into the spacious lot. "Do you think this is good, or should I park over in that spot?" I ask inanely.

"I don't know," Mom says. "You know what you're doing. I don't know."

"I don't usually know what I'm doing, but I pretend," I say, smiling. But it's a mirthless joke. I do know what I'm doing. I know exactly what I'm doing.

Mom goes into the facility easily, to see her "new apartment" as we have named it, and to see if Perry Como might be there. She notices her name on the door of her assigned room and, seeing her picture of Perry lying on a bed by the window (as we have arranged with the staff), fairly runs into the room, grabs the picture, and holds it to her with breathless excitement. The social worker points to a vase on the night table.

"Look at the flowers Perry left for you," she says. "He's never done that before."

Mom also responds positively to two young female aides and, while they and Perry Como hold her attention, Wayne and I recede into the background. With a behind-the-back wave of her hand, the social worker signals us to leave and we literally run down the hall to the Unit exit door. Just as we reach it we hear Mom's voice. "Terry! Terry!" Her tone is insistent, frantic, and more than tinged with fear. We are in pretty bad shape ourselves as the door closes and locks behind us. We peer through the little window, but Mom doesn't come out of her room and we hear no more.

We go out to the car, then return, certain that by now she is in a terrible state. Again we peek in. Nothing. We find a nurse, vent our fear and guilt to her for ten minutes while she listens patiently and offers quiet, detached assurance.

We ride home through vernal streets, every unfurling leaf along the roadsides affirming hope and new life. I stop at our mail service, but instead of getting out to retrieve the mail, Wayne bursts into tears.

On this fine, fresh spring afternoon we echo one another with great, wracking sobs, and fall into each other's arms.

17

"There's no one there to care."

—Helen

May 10, Year Two I miss Mom. Wayne misses Mom. Meg, manager of the Secure Unit, encourages me to visit and I do, but it's not the same as when she lived with us. I don't know if I'll ever have the same feeling. We don't live there. It's a facility. The staff have been welcoming, and that's helpful, but there's no place for us there, no structure within which we can just "be" together. There's no "Good morning," no running into each other about the house, no sharing of meals, no "Good night." Good times or bad, life unfolds spontaneously when people live together. A visit is just a visit.

Twenty-four hours a day was too much, but we didn't want it reduced to near-zero. We couldn't find another choice, one that would give us our lives and Mom, too.

May 19 I'm worried about my mother's physical health. Her feet are swollen, there are red marks on her legs, she's not sleeping at night, and she's so tired she can barely walk. But she smiles at people and seems slowly to be gaining some level of comfort with the residents, staff, and physical surroundings.

Mom and I sing old songs while I put up her hair. In between, she asks me about Wayne. "How did the two of you get so close?" she wants to know.

"Well, we've known each other a long time. We're married now," I say as though catching up news for an old friend.

"That's good."

"You know what, Mom? Wayne thinks of you as his mom, too. Like he has two mothers."

She smiles. "I'm just happy that you're happy," she says.

"You always were like that."

"Well, of course. I'm your mother."

May 20 Every time we enter or leave the Unit we necessarily go through the locked door. Often, Terry's mother is with us. She seems to know that this is the way out, but cannot find the "open sesame" to accomplish it for herself.

A keyless entry box activated by a simple code hangs on the wall next to the door, fully accessible not only to staff and visitors but equally so to every resident. No resident knows how to work it, and my sense is that none sees any connection between this box and opening the door. For her part, Mom has developed a ritual of licking her finger and smearing it in various mysterious configurations on the small window set into the door, but has not yet found freedom by this method.

Today she instructs me in her escape methodology: "Do like this," she says, moving her hands in tight circles in front of the door, "until something happens." While she speaks I punch in the release code. She finishes, I finish, the door swings open, and Mom's face lights with surprise and glee. But not inquisitiveness. Nothing for the future.

"That's my car," she says, spotting the Subaru in the lot once we are outside.

"It'll be there whenever you need it, Mom."

"Okay. You just let me know when."

May 21 "How are you feeling?" I ask my mother as we sit together in the Unit's sunny courtyard.

She gazes at the cobalt-blue Colorado sky beyond the high fence. "I don't feel good at all," she says.

"Why?"

"Because I don't know where the hell I am." She pauses. "There's no one there to care."

June 3 Wayne and I had been visiting Mom every other day. Then last week I came five days in a row. We went out a lot: shopping, visiting friends, a snack at a café. I hoped that this would be a way to have a more normal relationship with her, but each day she seemed more restless and uncomfortable during these excursions. Nor did she want to return to the nursing home.

Leaving continues to be difficult. Sometimes Mom grabs onto me and won't let go. Once she spit at me. It haunts me to think that this may never change.

I think what I have to do is deepen our relationship, move it to a more essential level.

June 7 We had the 30-day Staffing this week to review Mom's "fit" for the Unit. The staff reported positive things and mentioned no negatives beyond normal adjustment issues. Their recommendation is that Mom stay, and Wayne and I concur. It feels like a milestone has been passed, like Mom lives there now.

June 21 My mother is often soiled and smelly when I come to visit. It upsets me terribly to find her in this condition, to have to get her cleaned up before we do anything else. To know that she lives like this. "They've got me locked up in here," she told me yesterday.

June 22 Today Wayne and I take her out for ice cream, but she won't get out of the car. When we return to Holly Hills, again she refuses to get out. "You go in and do your business," she says. "It's not our business, Mom. We're at your place. You're home," he tells her, and I can hear the exasperation in his tone. He thinks she's upset about being back, that she's resisting, but I don't think that's it. I think she doesn't recognize this place.

* * * * *

This is something I have to remind myself of—or be reminded of by Terry—constantly: although *I* recognize Holly Hills each time I pull into the parking lot and see the familiar façade of the building, I can't assume that Mom does. Not even when I hear her read the big sign.

But even if I can learn this lesson, what does it portend for the future? In almost every instance in which I speak to someone I presume that the two of us share a multitude of skills and understandings—language, history, identity, memory, vocabulary and rules of grammar, even moment-by-moment sensory experience. As Mom's dementia deepens, how will we communicate, and about what? What is to become of our relationship?

June 26   I've come to wash and set Mom's hair, a task I've performed for her for almost two years. "Boy," she says when I arrive, "I was just about to call Wayne to come and do it!" This strikes me as funny: Wayne has never done her hair; nor, I think, would she let him if he tried.

After I finish and Mom and I are on our way back to the Unit, she points to her soft and shiny locks with pride and tells the first person she sees, "Wayne did my hair."

June 27   Always a good speller and avid letter writer, my mother-in-law recently signed a card to her granddaughter's little boy "Grate Grandma."

She rarely writes anything anymore. Perhaps she can't think what to say, and also, I suspect, she is losing the complex motor skills that writing requires. But it is also true that she has no real opportunity to write. No writing materials, no encouragement, no need or reason. Because of her illness, we and others have for two years steadily taken over her responsibilities and, our good intent notwithstanding, her contact with the outside world has steadily diminished. Her dementia furthers her dementia.

June 30 As I skim through my journal of these past two years of my mother's illness, I come across the words "just love her" scattered through.

I keep forgetting that. It's so simple and elegant, yet I lose track of it again and again. When it does come to me, as now, it's a new insight each time, and hits me with the force of a blow.

July 7 My mother-in-law is wandering in and out of other residents' rooms, dressed in another resident's clothes which are two sizes too small. She smells soiled.

"Helen is being difficult," an aide tells me. "She needs a shower. She shouldn't leave the Unit until she gets one."

Eventually she and another aide and I convince Mom to take a shower, with my promise of a walk afterward clinching the deal. I am both a participant and cheerleader in the shower preparations, until Mom gets stripped to her waist. "Wayne's never seen me like this," she says and I volunteer to wait outside. Laughter emanates from the stall from all three of them, interspersed with angry shouts from Mom—"Don't do that. Stop it. Don't *do* that!"—followed by more laughter.

Mom asks me to come in again. It's a large shower stall, big enough for her in the wheeled shower chair, the two aides and myself, with extra space for clothing, towels, and shampoo. Mom is soaped from head to foot, mildly restrained in the chair by one aide holding her hands, partly for Mom's safety and partly to prevent her from swinging out at them when she doesn't understand, or just doesn't want, what is being done. She objects the most strongly to touch and washing of her buttocks and groin.

I decide my job is to stand in the corner and smile. I tell her a story Terry has often told me, about Russ drying Terry so vigorously when she was a child that she thought he would take her skin off. Mom seems to remember. She emerges from the shower relaxed and comfortable.

July 25 A few days ago our visit was very discouraging in every respect. When we arrived she was soiled; many of her basic possessions, including her shoes, could not be found; we learned that she had been excluded from an outing earlier in the day, for reasons we never were able to clarify; and she was ill at ease when we took her out for a ride with us.

But today everything is different. She is bowled over with excitement and joy, and her enthusiastic, positive mood carries through the entire visit. We attend a music presentation together, sitting on either side of her, she squeezing Wayne's and my hands in rhythm to the music.

August 7, Year Three We go into the Staffing, the first we've been invited to since June, with some anxiety. Terry and I don't want to appear critical of the staff or alienate them in any way, but we want to deal with what we feel are important issues in this formal forum. One is Mom's hygiene, or lack of it, and what can be done to improve the situation. Another is that her personal belongings are frequently missing, and that when we raise these concerns with the staff their perpetually low-key response runs along the lines of "We'll keep an eye out for them." We understand that the residents, Mom included, are confused and that they move things around pretty freely, but after all is said and done, Mom needs her eyeglasses and her shoes. And it isn't only she and the other residents who misplace her things. We frequently find other residents' clothing hanging neatly in her closet, placed there, we feel certain, by staff.

We go in with these concerns, but the Activities Director says that Mom is getting along with people, that the residents like her and welcome her, and that she participates in most activities. Meg, the Unit manager, is bubbly and quite positive about her, although one remark in passing, that Mom has been less combative, throws me a bit. I don't think I've ever heard that word used by this staff about her, although they have occasionally told us of mildly negative behaviors on her part. Once, she threw a glass of water on someone.

I saw her swat at the staff during the shower I helped with a month ago, probably not an isolated incident, and a month before that, in a pique of anger about Terry's leaving, she spit on her. She can be verbally coarse. All this I know, but "combative" seems to me too strong, a different thing altogether. It is not as though this is a point that Meg has raised for discussion, however. It is just a word she has chosen to use—a negative word to my ear, but one used in a friendly tone and an overall positive context—and before I can digest it or respond, the subject has long passed.

All the staff who are present seem so genuinely interested in Mom and good-willed toward her that I, and Terry too, apparently, find it easy to soften our agenda, to pass over a few things and to trust that improvement is on the way. There are imperfections in their system, but the staff seem well-intentioned and tolerant. They tell us that showering and personal hygiene are the most difficult for them in working with Mom, but that any resulting upsets are transitory, and she is on an even keel afterward.

August 12 I'm washing and putting up my mother's hair, one of our familiar and favorite shared activities.

Mom: I never expected to see you today.

Terry: No, you didn't know I was coming. So what have you been doing?

M: Nothing.

T: Nothing?

M: Except worrying.

T: I wish you wouldn't worry. You know we're taking care of things.

M: I know we are. I know *you* are.

T: Yeah. We all are. You're taking care of what you can take care of, and I'm taking care of what I can take care of, and Sharon's taking care of what she can take care of. Wayne's taking care of what he can take care of (laughs).

M: (sounding rather pleased) So I'm being taken care of.

T: Yeah. And you're taking care of things, too.

M: When I get home I'm gonna look silly. 'Cause I'm not used to having my hair up.

T: (laughs) You're going to look terrific! . . . So what's new? Did you see Lawrence Welk?

M: No. I don't get to see things like that. You know, they come on with other, like other things, and I miss it.

T: Oh, I'm sorry.

M: Wayne couldn't come today, huh?

T: Yeah, he's going to come. He had to get some things in the mail and call some schools. But he'll be here in a little while.

M: I sure didn't expect you today.

T: I know. You never know when to expect me. . . . I get to surprise you!

M: Yeah. . . . I'm gonna have to get my hair curled.

T: I'm curling it right now. . . . I'm cutting it and curling it both. . . . Let's sing. (sings) *Every time it rains it rains . . .*

M: *. . . pennies from heaven.*

T & M: *Did you know each cloud contains, pennies from heaven?*

M: *You'll find your fortune falling, all over town. Be sure that your umbrella is upside down.* Now what comes?

T: *Trade them for a . . .*

T & M: *. . .package of sunshine and flowers.*

T: *If you want the things you love, you've gotta have . . .*

T & M: *. . . showers. So when you hear it thunder, don't run under a tree.*

T: *There'll be . . .*

T & M: *. . . pennies from heaven for you and for me.*

T: I like that song. You taught it to me. It was the first song you sang in a night club. The audience threw pennies onto the stage, and you were afraid they didn't like you. Then you realized they were showing their appreciation, for the song and the singer.

M: (Nods, smiling. She begins humming, then picks up the words) *. . . all over town.*

T & M: *Be sure that your umbrella is upside down.*

T: *Trade them for a package of . . .*

M: Are you sure you have everything now?

T: Yeah. . . . *sunshine and flowers. If you want the things you love . . .*

T & M: *. . . you must have showers. So . . .*

M: *. . . when you hear it thunder, don't run under a tree. There'll be pennies from heaven for you and for me.*

T: Okay!

M: Well, I'm sorry that Wayne hasn't been here.

T: Yeah, he'll be here pretty soon, though.

M: Oh, will he?

T: Yes.

M: Will he know where to go?

T: Oh yeah. I told him I was going to be doing your hair.

M: Oh.

T: So he knows where.

M: Oh, God. . . . This is one thing I did not expect.

T: I know. I'm always surprising you.

M: Yeah.

T: Maybe I should call you before I come. Would that be better?

M: No. No, surprising me is better.

T: (laughs) Okay.

M: *So when you hear it thunder, don't climb under a tree. There'll be pennies from heaven for you and for me.* I sure didn't expect you today.

T: (laughs) I know. I surprised you!

M: I can't get over this, that you're here!

August 28   Sharon and Mom's great-grandson David have flown here to visit Mom on her eightieth birthday.

I go ahead to get her ready and we go out to wait for Wayne, Sharon, and David. Mom sits bolt upright, refusing to let herself lean against the bench back. She doesn't volunteer any knowledge of it being her birthday but I think she does know, either about her birthday or about the special visitors soon to arrive, because she studies every car and van that passes and talks about "after they come."

When they come up the walk she is thrilled to see them. She smiles every time she looks at David. We go to KFC. We give her all her presents and she especially likes David's—a brightly colored teddy bear—which she kisses and holds on to. At an ice cream shop Mom refuses to get out of the car at first but goes in with only a little coaxing, orders a huge butter pecan waffle cone, and devours the whole thing. She is completely at ease with Sharon and David. Their presence seems to calm her.

When we return to Holly Hills the very nice day begins to unravel. Mom doesn't want anything: not special attention, not cake, not the seat of honor, not a birthday song. "You'll have to get home on your own," she says, and we take this as our exit cue.

On the way out, David correctly enters the door code on the key pad, despite the fact that he had no explanation or instruction and only one observation when we came in.

August 30 Mom sits on her bed, surrounded by cards, her birthday photo album, her teddy bear. There are no sheets on the bed. She smells of feces. She says she's not feeling well, that her head hurts. I can see the veins protruding above her temple, and her eyelids are swollen and red. She lies down on her bed, something she has never done before when Wayne and I are here.

Wayne turns off the overhead fluorescent and we sing to her softly in the subdued light. I stroke her head. She quiets, relaxes, accepts our nurturing. Although we were concerned before coming about "Where are Sharon and David?" questions, there are none.

Suddenly Mom sits up. "Let's go home!" she says. She rises from the bed, gathers up all her cards, the album, and her bear.

"Let's go," I agree.

Mom smears on the glass while Wayne keys the code, the door swings open, and out we go, not home but into the flower garden. We make a slow circuit of the yard, oohing and ahhing to one another about the flowers and ornaments along the path. Mom has entirely forgotten about going home. The words were important at the moment she uttered them, but I have come to learn that they convey an emotional rather than a literal meaning. Home is no longer a place but a concept. Speaking the word and taking action—any action—gives her comfort. I am able to respond with enthusiasm because I don't fear anymore that she's expecting a certain thing to happen.

As we approach the Unit doors, Wayne and I execute the perfect, instinctive choreography—one we've never actually discussed or planned—which we've been using for some time to avoid the pain of Mom separating from me. I simply stop in my tracks, slipping silently out of sight while Wayne deftly steps into my position beside Mom. I remain outside the Unit. Mom and Wayne walk inside. She never notices my disappearance or mentions my name. Today our maneuver is again a success, though, as always, a bittersweet one.

I peer through the small window and watch Wayne and Mom recede down the long hall. They come upon Frances, a verbally noncommunicative resident only recently admitted. Mom reaches out, in that very physical way she has of relating to the world, and strokes Frances's hair lightly. "Your hair looks very nice," she tells her.

"Hi, Helen!" It's an aide, Kristen, smiling and welcoming her.

Mom surges forward. Wayne falls away like a spent booster rocket, then turns back toward me as my mother disappears around the corner.

18

I can imagine few settings that better reveal the nature of
psychological stress than a nursing home.

—Robert M. Sapolsky

September 6, Year Three The Holly Hills social worker
called this morning and told us that my mother is behaving aggressively on the Unit and that this is a matter of concern to the staff. A
meeting is scheduled for the 10th to discuss options.

We come to see Mom this afternoon, partly in response to this
morning's call, worried about what we will see. But there is no
problem during the time that we are here. Everything seems fine.

September 9 Mom is tranquil and easy-going the whole time I
am on the Unit this evening.

September 10 The staff describe Mom as aggressive and agitated
and say that this has increased recently, although Terry and I are not
aware that there has been any serious on-going problem to begin
with. The main source of conflict seems to center on Mom's bowel
incontinence and difficulties the staff have in working with her in
relation to that. Recommendations resulting from the meeting
include treatment of a current urinary tract infection, use of a stool
bulking agent, and putting Mom on a toileting program to prevent
soiling.

After the meeting I decide to visit Mom on the Unit. Peering
through the window before opening the door, I observe her and
Frances, arm in arm, walking quietly down the corridor together.
Another resident, Agnes, approaches from the dining area and al-

most immediately a fight erupts between her and Mom. Two aides quickly appear and separate the two. Mom goes into her room.

When I enter the Unit, Mom spots me immediately and greets me warmly. She clutches a bed pillow against her upper body. As we pass Agnes in the hallway, Agnes crouches, like a fighter in the ring, and wags her finger upward at Mom. "I hate you," she says. "You're hideous. I want you to be dead." The words burst from her mouth, snapping like tiny firecrackers in the space between us. The display is so unexpected and extreme, yet emanates from a body so ancient, contorted, and small, that I find myself torn between laughter and genuine, if momentary, fear. Mom pushes Agnes's arm aside and sticks her tongue out at her. Agnes swings, kicks at her, and continues her verbal assault. I step between them. Agnes strikes me in the jaw with her tiny fist. The entire exchange lasts less than fifteen seconds. Again staff appear just at the end.

Mom and I take a walk outside in the courtyard and I can feel the tension in her grip on my hand. She shows me a blood blister and several scratch marks on her right forearm. They are not from the immediate scuffle, but they are fresh. They weren't there when I visited last evening.

When we re-enter the building Agnes again lashes out verbally. I keep my body between them and no physical exchange takes place.

At Mom's request we leave the Unit and go for a half-mile walk, long by her standards. She maintains an outwardly positive demeanor, but her conversation is more rudimentary than usual, her responses and smile forced and mechanical. She still holds her pillow like a shield across her midsection. "I need it," she says when I offer to carry it for her.

September 13   Terry's mother is sitting in the Day Area, chatting with another resident.

I talk briefly with one of the nursing staff, Trish, who seems to have many good ideas about how to work with Mom. She gave her a shower last night and, while she does not suggest that it was an easy task, gives no impression that it was anything out of the ordinary in her experience with residents generally. She says positive things about Mom, both as a person and as a resident with whom she has many interactions.

I am surprised, therefore, to hear that when the doctor came today, she and the staff agreed that the problems Terry and I first heard complaint of on September 6 are continuing, difficult, and unimproved. They have decided, short of our flat refusal to permit it, to start her on a new medication, Inderal. Our understanding is that it will be used, along with the buspirone which Mom has remained on since early spring, to decrease anxiety. Although our first choice would be behavioral intervention, this medication approach is the preference of doctor and staff at this time. Perhaps it will prove helpful. We decide to allow it.

September 14   One of the nurses, Janice, calls to say that my mother slapped her while she was trying to get her to swallow her pills with water instead of chewing them. She is making a report of the incident as legally required, she tells me. And she is calling us, she says, also as required. She tells me she is sorry to bother me. "Is there anything I can do?" I ask. "No," she says, "she's fine now. She had a good day."

This is the first such "required" call we have received since Mom's admission to the Unit.

* * * * *

Today I submitted for inclusion in my mother-in-law's file a write-up of my observation of the interactions between her and Agnes on September 10, followed by these reflections:

> . . . [T]here may be circumstances entirely external to Helen . . . which directly affect her emotional state and consequent behavior. If the full precipitating event(s) is not observed by staff, as in the above-described instances, Helen's tension or

anger directed at others later on may appear irrational and unprovoked. Today, had she not been
able to "take control" of her situation by getting off
the Unit and getting some significant physical exercise, had she instead been required to behave in a
more specific, staff-directed way, I think she may
well have acted out. Perhaps this happened anyway
later in the day, as it was apparent to me when I
departed that there was still residual tension in her
from the earlier interactions with Agnes.

The truth is, *I* had some residual effect; *I* tensed
a little as we re-entered the Unit and neared Agnes's door. How much more so Helen, who can
feel just as much, but can comprehend, express,
and influence so much less than I?

September 15 It's almost comfy in Mom's room today. She sits
in the chair, I behind her, combing her hair, while Wayne is perched
on the bed, sorting through all her clothes and belongings, marking
and re-marking them with a laundry pen as necessary.

"How many kids do you have?" I ask her.

"Three."

Since she has only two I'm curious to explore further. "What are
their names?" Mom has no idea. "Well, there's me!" I say with enthusiasm.

"Yeah!" she says, and it brings it home to me that, while she
clearly "knows" us, she may not know for certain anymore who
Wayne and I are. Not all the time. But it doesn't matter to her,
because she's very close to us, and that's what she does know all the
time.

"I'm putting my mom's name in this book," Wayne says to no
one in particular as he prints her name on her photo album.

It catches me, touches me, that no sooner has my mother told
me that she has three unnameable kids, than Wayne—possessed of
a perfectly good mother of his own—should refer to her as "my
mom."

Maybe she's more in tune than I know.

September 16 Mom has just finished supper and is sitting quietly at the table. I speak briefly with an aide, who says that she is doing much better, that her behavior is much improved. Mom herself is in a good mood. The staff seem at ease with her. A fine visit.

Only later does Terry tell me that, minutes after my talk with the aide, she received a report from Janice that it had been a fairly difficult day with Mom, that there had been "some incidents."

September 17 The social worker calls this afternoon, telling me there are "more concerns with your Mom" and that "she is very aggressive" toward other residents and staff. She describes a situation in which my mother told Cleo, while in Cleo's room—which was also Mom's room for a time—to "get out." When Cleo refused, the social worker reports, Mom "swatted the air." She calls my mother "a danger" and "unmanageable." She wants a medical evaluation.

Wayne and I are confused. With few exceptions—Wayne's experience with Mom and Agnes last week being the most notable—we've always seen neutral to positive interactions between Mom and people on the Unit. "She's different when you're here," they tell us.

Is she? And, if so, why? What is different when we are not present? Something is going on, and we want to understand what that might be. Wayne's background in psychology and education have given him experience in objective observation and recording of behavior. We decide that he will go immediately to Holly Hills to observe without interacting with my mother. To be there, as best he can, without being there.

* * * * *

I arrive at 4:30 p.m., stop briefly at the social worker's office to inform her of my purpose, then enter the Unit to find Mom sitting in a common spot for her, a kind of love seat located next to the nursing station. Cleo sits next to her and they appear to be talking quietly. As soon as she sees me, Mom comes over and greets me. "I can't visit right now," I tell her. "I'm working."

She accepts this readily and tells me that she's "going upstairs." It's something I've heard her, and other residents of this single-story building, say before; and it brings me an internal smile as I watch her stroll up the hall, check the Unit doors briefly and, to my surprise, key the pad, although without result.

The social worker comes onto the Unit and she and Mom share a few friendly words before Mom continues on her way. She spots Cleo again, and waves to her. Also to another resident and a staff member who are entering the Unit.

She heads back to the two-seater couch, which is occupied now by Aubrey, a nurse, who appears to be doing some sort of paperwork. Mom stoops to pick up some manila folders which lie on the seat next to Aubrey. She sits down, holding the items now on her lap. With some urgency in her voice, Aubrey asks Mom for the folders, reaching for them as she speaks. "No," Mom says, just as urgently, and appears to tighten her hold. The interaction quickly intensifies, with Aubrey variously demanding ("Give it to me"), explaining ("Those are very important papers"), and coaxing ("How about we trade? You give me those papers, and I'll give you this magazine"). But Mom is not persuaded. "You are going to give them back," Aubrey says with finality and a brief tug-of-war ensues. Aubrey ends up with her papers, Mom with the magazine.

She remains seated for a minute or two, looking about the room with a pleasant expression on her face, then gets up and approaches me. "Wayne, come upstairs with me," she asks.

"I can't, Mom. I'm working," I tell her again. She sticks out her tongue and blows noisy air at me in the traditional "raspberry," and goes up the hall alone.

When she returns, she heads again to the love seat. Aubrey is still there, her materials again resting on the vacant seat. Mom bends to pick them up. The nurse grabs for them, and whether she gets to them first or snatches them from Mom's hands, I cannot tell. Mom swats Aubrey on the upper body/arms with the magazine Aubrey gave her a few minutes ago. "Please don't hit me, Helen," Aubrey says. There is a brief further verbal exchange which I cannot hear and Mom sits down.

By 5:10 Mom is seated alone when Kristen approaches and asks if she may sit next to her. Mom agrees, but appears disinterested. "Where's Becky?" the aide asks, referring to Mom's favorite staff member. When Mom does not respond, Kristen repeats her question. "I don't *know!*" Mom snaps.

Soon after, Kristen and Aubrey decide that Mom is "poopy" and Kristen invites Mom to "get cleaned up." Mom refuses. Now the aide asks Mom if she would like to go for a walk. "For a walk, yes," she replies. They start off down the hall, but as they approach Mom's room Kristen and another staff member physically guide her, Mom resisting, through the doorway of her room, and then, more forcibly, into the bathroom. Aubrey joins them. I move closer. The door is mostly closed but I can hear Mom cursing and demanding to be left alone. Suddenly I see her face, her eyes seeing me through the crack at the hinge side of the door. "My son-in-law is out there!" she exclaims, and I quickly move out of her line of sight.

"I don't want you in there!" she shouts at them a moment later, little doubt in my mind as to what she refers.

"Please don't hit, Helen." A staff member's voice.

"I'm going to hit until you're dead," Mom tells her.

Five long minutes pass, after which the nurse suggests that some staff should leave. Mom agrees. Aubrey encourages that Mom "dismiss" the two aides, which she does. "You can stay," she tells Aubrey.

As dinner approaches, several requests are made for Mom to come to the table, but she refuses. When Kristen again invites her, Mom hits at her. "No I am *not* going to sit down," she says. "Sit on your own ass."

A few minutes later an aide brings Mom's food to her on a tray. Aubrey asks her if she is going to eat.

"No."

"Well, will you take your medicine, your pills?" Aubrey asks.

"No."

"Do you want some water?"

"No. Kiss my ass."

A few minutes later Kristen invites Mom to eat or to have some juice.

"No," she says, sticking out her tongue.

"Here's your Jell-O, Helen," Kristen says.

"I don't care what the hell it is."

Hardly a minute later, Kristen says to Mom, "Helen, the nurse wanted you to come and talk to her."

"Kiss my ass," Mom tells her.

Aubrey says, "Helen, Terry brought you these pills." Mom says nothing, but retreats quickly to her room. Aubrey follows her, uses a similar coax, and Mom takes the medications.

At 5:50 Mom still has not eaten anything. Kristen and Aubrey enter her room to get her changed into night clothes. Mom resists. "Why do you want to get your way?" she wants to know. "I'm just trying to help you," Kristen says. "I don't want them on, goddammit!" Mom tells her.

Kristen leaves and Mom comes out with a pajama top and robe over slacks. The staff tell her she is only half changed and urge her to change into her pajama bottoms.

Mom approaches me now, wants me to go with her. I tell her I can't. "Shit on you," she says and returns to her room. Two of the staff now enter her room and forcibly take her into the bathroom to change her slacks for pajamas. There follows fifteen minutes of arguing and yelling. The following remarks are representative:

Staff: Helen, stop, please. Let her get your bottoms off.

Mom: I don't need any help, goddammit!

S: Don't hit her, please.

M: I can button my own blouses!

S: Don't kick.

M: You're a horse's ass, too.

S: Let's pee.

M: God damn son-of-a-bitch! I want my clothes *on*.

Twenty-five minutes after staff leave Mom's room she has not yet emerged. It has been two hours since my arrival. I abandon my observer status—I have seen plenty—and go to her room. She is lying on her bed.

"Well, did you get anything accomplished?" she asks, in apparent reference to my "work."

"I think so," I tell her. "There's more to do, but I can finish it later." She is wide awake, and happy for contact with me. When she asks about a commotion in the hallway I tell her, "They're playing some kind of game, I think." Mom is eager to join.

Many residents and several staff are in the hall. Mom smiles at everyone and quickly becomes a part of the game. When Agnes makes a sudden face at Mom she sticks her tongue out at her in response. A male aide steps between them, facing my mother-in-law. "We have to let everyone have a turn," he tells her in a gentle yet chiding tone.

Mom initiates interactions marked by affectionate touch and speech with two other residents, and is actively and positively involved with everyone she sees, staff and residents, for the better part of an hour. She goes into Cleo's room as Cleo is getting ready for bed. I stand unseen nearby, listening for five minutes to their amiable, confused conversation as they sit together on Cleo's bed.

By 7:30 she is tired. Three times she lets me tuck her into bed, then immediately gets up—positive, smiling, and alert. A few minutes later I'm waiting in the hall to see if she has settled in when Kristen enters her room. A brief, friendly exchange floats through the doorway.

I leave for home, my pocket full of notes, my heart full of questions.

September 18 Mom's doctor called at the house while Wayne was at Holly Hills last evening. She told me that she was given an ultimatum by some unnamed—to me, at least—person at Holly

Hills: my mother must either be hospitalized for an evaluation, be placed immediately on a major tranquilizer—thioridazine—or we must move her out of Holly Hills. She didn't like that they went through her rather than us. Nor did I.

When she calls again this morning, Wayne summarizes for her his observations of last evening. The three of us discuss the hospitalization alternative, which I don't want, given Mom's experiences in California last spring. Besides, it would insert a new doctor into the mix, one not chosen by us but who, for all practical and perhaps legal purposes, would have primary-physician authority.

The doctor assures us that she can handle supervision of a thioridazine regimen for Mom at Holly Hills, and also says that she will call the nursing home "to see if there is any leeway" in their position. We tell her that we prefer increasing the Inderal to starting on thioridazine.

I went to bed last night with the conscious intention of learning something in the night about what would be best for Mom. I had a dream, about a "fish out of water." One interpretation seems obvious: Mom is in the wrong place, one where she can't survive. But Wayne suggests to me another. She needs nourishment where she is, he says. She needs water—love and caring—poured on her *here*, not to be picked up and thrown into a pool somewhere else.

Maybe so. But I think they simply don't want her. Part of me wants to go over there this minute, take Mom by the hand, walk out that door, and never come back.

* * * * *

Meg calls around noon. She is well aware of the "three options" and encourages us to talk to Mom's doctor. I tell her about how the phone call from the social worker on September 6 came at Terry and me from out of the blue, and that we've felt one step behind ever since. "We've tried to respond in helpful ways," I say, "but we wonder if you and the staff perceive us as unhelpful." "Oh, no," Meg assures me. I talk generally, no names or specific incidents, about the events of last evening, and offer to share my observations with her. "I think they're worthwhile," I tell her, and emphasize that we want to keep open lines of communication with all the staff. "We want to be helpful to you. We're working toward the same goal," I tell her. She is full of praise for everything I say. I tell her that Terry and I would rather go with Inderal than the thioridazine. She says she'll check out that possibility.

Just before three, the Holly Hills administrator calls. Seems like suddenly we're on everybody's call list. Her name is Betty. She speaks in a casual, friendly tone, which makes me ill at ease, as we do not have a casual, friendly relationship. We have no relationship at all. I do not remember that she has ever introduced herself or spoken to Terry or to me in the 4½ months Mom has been living at her nursing home. When the conversation begins covering some of the same ground I just spoke with Meg about two hours ago I ask if she realizes that Meg and I have talked. Yes, she does, and now her message becomes more pointed, and discouraging.

On the one hand she insists on a course of thioridazine if Mom is to stay, while on the other she describes the severe risks of the drug and says that it's very difficult to find a therapeutic dosage. She tells me "the other families are complaining" about Mom, and that her staff is, too. "This is our first job," she says, "to make sure that people are safe."

I tell her that in Mom's 4½ months at Holly Hills neither Terry nor I have seen her attack a resident or initiate any real aggression against anyone without provocation. I mention several recent incidents with Agnes, including the one last night, as examples. "We track all these things," she says. I tell her that in the incidents involving Mom and other residents which I have witnessed, the staff did not see the provocations but only Mom's response, and may have tracked them incorrectly. I tell her that I observed things last night that could have been handled differently. I suggest an increase in Inderal which, in addition to being more benign, seems preferable also because Mom already has an existing blood level.

"It has to be thioridazine," Betty says. "We just can't experiment."

But getting the dosage right, isn't that experimentation? She says that she will have to bring in extra staff to sit with Mom during an adjustment period to the thioridazine. Why not bring in extra staff to sit with her while they increase the Inderal? Better yet, why not bring in extra staff for the sake of better coverage? Maybe *that* will solve the problem.

My sense, one which has grown with each passing minute, is that Betty has called only to get Mom out of her facility or onto thioridazine. One of these two.

My son-in law is out there! Mom's words from yesterday haunt my memory. A simple statement of fact? Embarrassment? Or was it a call for assistance? *My son-in-law is out there. He won't let you do this to me!*

If it was the latter, I'm sorry, Mom. In the interest of dispassionate, objective observation, I did. But what about today? What keeps me from telling Betty now, not about Mom and Agnes, not about things that could have been handled differently, but precisely and in detail about her own staff's behaviors? Simply this: I have no confidence that Betty and I are having a genuine discussion. We are not teammates, I fear, but adversaries, in a contest whose outcome was determined before the opening bell. And if I am right, if I should dare now to refuse all three of her options, take the offensive on Mom's behalf and fail, what then? Am I prepared to go over there and get her? As though we have another place for her to go?

"Nobody wants her," I cry into the phone, the words no sooner past my lips than I am mortified by them, embarrassed to have turned to her, of all people, for comfort.

"Oh no," Betty protests. "She's so sweet." Jagged glass.

My vision just a few weeks ago was that this is the place where Mom will live out her life. All along we've been urged to let go, to live our own lives and do our work, to trust them to take care of her. I'd begun to believe it, to settle into it.

I ask Betty for a few hours to consider our decision. "No," she says, "I've promised the other residents' families." Who are these families? Has any complaint actually been made? For one brief moment I fantasize sleuthing the truth out, interrogating the families and all the staff, finding out the "real" story. It's preposterous, I know. And, ultimately, what is the point? What do we gain for Mom if we succeed in forcing her on them?

I can think of nothing else to do, nothing more to say. Betty's silent waiting smothers and exhausts me, and I am filled with fear.

"Okay," I tell her. "Go ahead with the thioridazine."

Fear, and now shame.

September 19 "Wayne!" Mom calls out immediately when I arrive, then takes me by the arm and leads me around the Unit like a manic tour guide. The drug's effect, or Mom's response to it, or some combination of the two, seems paradoxical. She appears sedated, almost stuporous, yet she is not calm. She is active, on her feet, and seems agitated, as though some part of her being realizes that her capabilities are diminished and has decided that she must make up the difference through sheer effort. Her lids droop but the eyes are scanning, searching, and when words come they pour from her mouth like wet cement, full of potential but ill-formed. "I doan like the way thozh people are lookin' at ush," she says, indicating everyone in sight and no one at all. "Like they wanna shteal somethin'." Her grip on my arm is strong.

But for all her energy, her steps are small and feeble and her feet do not quite keep pace with her intentions. She doesn't have a good sense of her body in space, wobbling occasionally and leaning forward when she walks, as though she battles a head wind. I don't see any tremors but her muscle tone is poor, her voice weak. Much of what I see reminds me of her condition the day she stepped off the plane 4½ months ago.

At the dinner table she is mostly disconnected from people and circumstance, reaching for whatever food is in sight, others' as well as her own. When soup is placed in front of her, she immediately puts a fork in the bowl and tries to feed herself.

I express concern about Mom's condition to the nurse. She responds by pointing out a woman unknown to me, the "extra staff person" it turns out, that Betty said they would provide. I had no idea she was present until this moment. She was not with Mom when I arrived and has not approached or introduced herself. Now, while Mom struggles with her soup and fork, she stands motionless across the room.

September 20 She's a little stronger and more alert than yesterday, though still walking in small steps, as though an invisible chain links her ankles. Her speech is still slurred (if 100 were normal, last night she was 15, this morning 40). "I didn't know anythin' yeshterday," she says, clutching my arm.

She tells me that she needs a bathroom, but in her present condition I am certain that she has no idea where any of the bathrooms on the Unit are located. I lead her to the one in her room, turn on the light in the windowless cubicle. She starts to slip her slacks down.

"Do you need any help?" I ask and wonder if she can hear my shyness.

She smiles sweetly and whispers in an appreciative yet private tone, "I can shit by myself, Wayne."

Afterward, moving slowly down the hall together, we approach Agnes, standing sentry just outside her room. Mom gives her a warm smile. Agnes contorts her face in reply. Mom sticks her tongue out at her.

"You're ugly," Agnes tells Mom. "You're stupid."

Again I am stung, but Mom seems more curious than insulted. "Why do you always . . .?" she starts, but cannot find the words to finish.

"You're almost as ugly as I am!" Agnes suddenly crows. Pleased with this joke on herself, she laughs and walks away.

———————

Terry's impression is that her mother has a lot of anger. "She may not be able to talk about it, or explain it even to herself, but she's not oblivious. She knows how she's being treated," Terry says, "and she doesn't like it. It's storing up, and it's going to come out. And when it does, it will have a lot to do with *their* behavior, how they've treated her. She is a *person*. She has feelings."

Aubrey was very positive about Mom today. She told me that she is "very manageable," as though this were a high compliment. It seems to me that manageability has lately become a major focus of the staff.

"This is a Special Care Unit!" Terry says. "She should be *allowed* to have her dementia. She shouldn't need to be as she would out in the world."

I can see the legitimacy of limits, even on a Special Care Unit. The problem I have is that the staff tend to put the burden of management on the resident, as though it's Mom's job to be manageable rather than theirs to manage. Skillfully, creatively, and lovingly.

September 21 Terry and I had an argument this morning. She was upset. I was upset. She called me a name. I got loud and vulgar. We went through two cycles of that, sandwiching an apology in between, then escalated into a third argument.

"Look at how we reacted," Terry said. "Name-called and disrespected, look how we responded. So why should anyone think that Mom doesn't have the same kinds of feelings?"

Yes. Or that they mightn't come out in unpredictable and "unprovoked" ways?

September 23 Terry and I bring her mother to meet the Long-Term Care Ombudsman, whom we've recently contacted with our concerns about the quality of care she is receiving. I bring the lady out to the car to meet Mom and, despite her considerable limitations right now, both disease- and drug-induced, Mom is quite gracious. For her part, the ombudsman is straightforward in explaining to her the advocacy services she can provide. I'm sure Mom follows none of it. "I could come and visit with you sometime," the ombudsman offers. "Where you live."

"No," Mom says quickly. The ombudsman rephrases, offers her services a second time. Mom hesitates, then smiles and tilts her head up toward this friendly, earnest stranger. "If Wayne and Terry say it's okay," she says.

Standing there in the parking lot, I am touched that she falls back on us so, relies on us to make the decisions of her life, depends on us to keep her safe. Touched, and terrified, too.

19

"It's like West Side Story *here."*

—Helen

September 27, Year Three "There's no excuse for blaming residents," the ombudsman tells Wayne and me in her office. As a result of her visit to the Unit several days ago she feels that there is, in fact, some identification of my mother as a problem.

"Helen is a little different than most residents on the Unit," she says. "She's more direct, less passive."

October 2 Mom walks in small, wobbly steps. Terry and I have seen residents with bruises and black eyes, apparently from falls. We're afraid we'll come in some day and that will be Mom's situation.

Still unresolved, in my mind, is the question of whether the staff's issues with Mom could have been handled—whether those in the future could be still—in a more skillful, more humane, and more effective way.

To a significant degree Mom has faded into the Unit. She's more like the other people there now.

October 5 Over the past month there's been a constant warring in me between guilt, anger, and reluctant acceptance that Terry and I can't make things work as well as we want them to and believe they could. It's hard to believe sometimes what is going on. All this turmoil generated by Mom's incontinence, and yet I notice again today something we have brought to the staff's attention before: there is no toilet paper in Mom's bathroom.

With the ombudsman's encouragement, a Staffing has been scheduled for October 8.

October 6   Night or day, whenever I'm awake and not focused on something else, thoughts of my mother at Holly Hills dominate my consciousness. That there might be something that she wants to communicate but can't express; that someone is treating her badly; that her reaching out to others is misinterpreted.
I feel so sad. I can't get past it.

October 7   Terry's dream:

There are rattlesnakes in my house, slithering everywhere across the floor, churning it to dirt. They hide, tunneling, covering themselves over with the dust. Soon the floor looks normal again and I don't notice, can't really tell that I have rattlesnakes under my feet.

Suddenly I'm on one with both feet, its cool, muscled length squirming beneath my bare skin. It's huge. It doesn't want me on it, doesn't like me interfering with it.

"You're the ones causing the trouble," I want to say, but don't because they don't hear and don't care. They only want me off of them.

So now I have to do all the work. I have to get off of this angry snake somehow without pressing on it. I can't, and even if I somehow manage to, what about the next time? I'll never be able to relax. I'll have to be vigilant. Always. It won't matter what I do, or how hard I try to do it right.

I'm going to get bitten.

October 8   On the surface there is openness and receptiveness on the part of Betty and all the staff who attend today's special Staffing on my mother-in-law. But it is a frustrating experience from the start.

No one is taking real charge of the meeting. People join the discussion at will and the focus drifts from one topic to another and from one individual's perspective to another's with little organized pursuit of any single issue. Nobody on staff seems to know how

Mom got on such a large initial dose of thioridazine. Trish says that there have been a lot of recent staff changes, and that some staff from other parts of the facility seem to view the Unit and its residents in a negative light. She says she's heard my mother-in-law's name mentioned specifically in this context. "The attitude around here has got to change," she adds. Betty declares, "I don't know what we have to offer Helen." Meg expresses frustration about the recent influx onto the Unit of residents in wheelchairs and with more severe disabilities than those admitted previously. Terry and I both voice our feeling that we and her mother have been betrayed by the events of the past month. "We just have to have better communication," Betty says.

Better communication? What Terry and I want is better care for her mother, better commitment to that goal, and a display of better skills in carrying out that commitment. When these things are in place I don't think communication will be an issue. Betty says that she wants to funnel all communications between us and Holly Hills through the Unit manager. "For consistency," she says. Better communication? More consistent communication? Fine. But the important communication is not between the staff and us. It's between the staff and Mom. We want better care.

October 9   My mother is overjoyed to see me. "I feel like I'm in a crazy house," she says. We go outside and she is talking to me the whole time. I can't make complete sense of it, but it's about how she has been trying to tell the staff here about something that upsets her. But what? For all her effort to tell me and to request my help, for all my burning desire to intercede for her, I cannot decode the specifics of her plea. But could it be that the specifics are not the heart of her message? Could it be that she is simply telling me, "I'm upset," that what she is asking for is nothing more than to be comforted?

"Don't worry, Mom," I tell her finally. "Let me tell them."

"Oh, good," she says, and real relief settles in her eyes and soothes her face.

At Kentucky Fried Chicken she moves slowly and seems sedated but has a good time anyway. She uses the toilet paper-equipped bathroom with no problem. We go to the grocery store and then to a friend's house to see her and her baby. Mom glows in their presence.

October 10   My mother-in-law is dozing in a chair at a table along the wall next to the two-seater couch. All the other residents and several staff are in the dining/day area. There are activities going on, both organized and spontaneous, and classical music plays in the background. This is a first, a far cry from the diet of pop/rock usually selected by the staff, and apparently a response to the fact that this issue, too, was raised at the Staffing two days ago.

Mom awakens and smiles at me and I sit next to her. She clutches a newspaper and several magazines in her arms, which are crossed and tight against her upper body. Mavis, a resident sitting at the same table, reaches for other papers on the tabletop. Mom tugs them from her, then plops them down again, closer to herself this time.

"Show me your rings, Mom," I say, hoping to turn her attention from Mavis. She smiles, splays the fingers of her left hand like a newlywed, turning the stones to the light. I admire them. "When Terry comes tomorrow, ask her to show you *her* rings," I say.

"Is she engaged now?"

"Yes, she is. In fact, we're married now!"

"You are?" she asks with surprise.

I hold out my hand for proof, showing her the wedding band Terry gave to me more than a quarter of a century ago.

"Good," she says.

Mavis reaches for the stack of newspapers. Again Mom yanks them away. "You can't have these," she tells her firmly. "These are mine." Mom picks up a flyswatter that has been lying on the table. My heart skips a beat.

To Mom's left sits Nola, 90+ years old, who seems oblivious to Mom and Mavis, but is very focused on Mavis's *chair*. She leans forward repeatedly, catching my eye when she can, and points to it in what seems to me a very mysterious fashion. I can see in Nola no response to the interaction between Mom and Mavis, nor sense any tension in her. Nevertheless, Mom turns to her and says reassuringly, "I won't hit you." And *my* tension level rises.

Mom abruptly rises from her seat and skillfully navigates the tight spaces between chairs, tables, wheelchairs, residents, and staff. As she passes Mary, a nurse who is putting up Bea's hair, Mary asks, "Do you need to go to the bathroom, Helen?" I neither hear nor see any response. "Do you need to go to the bathroom?" she says again, in an interested but otherwise neutral tone.

"Yes," Mom says.

"I'll come with you," she offers. Mom accepts, and they walk off arm in arm toward her room.

Nola, nimble and inquisitive as a schoolgirl, leans steeply in my direction and begins telling me about the chair. She thinks a strap is going to come undone and that Mavis might fall. I see now what she has been looking at. I study the situation, conclude that she is incorrect, and do my best to reassure her. She gets up and comes over next to me, scooting into the chair where Mom had been sitting.

"You missed your opportunity," she whispers.

"What do you mean?"

"She had to go somewhere."

At the very least I am curious. The whole time I thought she'd been obsessed with the chair! "What do you think she had to do?"

"She had to go to the pot," she answers gleefully.

"I think you're right. You're very observant."

I excuse myself to Nola, her face still lit with mystery and intrigue, and follow Mom and Mary's path, pausing outside Mom's bathroom door. I can hear both Mary's quiet voice, giving brief explanations and offers of assistance, and Mom's occasional responses. Although I cannot make out the words very well, I don't detect any trauma or upset in either voice. It sounds remarkably like a conversation.

I return to the dining room. Mom returns in a minute or two and sits down again, apparently relaxed and in a level mood; Mary picks up where she left off with Bea. When the opportunity presents itself I approach Mary. "How did that go?" I ask.

She looks at me with a puzzled expression. I mention the tales of woe I have heard over the past weeks.

"I've never had any problem with Helen," she says quietly. "You just have to be respectful." She puts her hand to her chest, spreading her fingers like a shield. "You know," she says in a voice that sounds like prayer, "she's very sensitive about this." She is facing Mom who is about ten feet away. I stand between them. We use my body as a screen to protect her from observing this reference to her mastectomies.

"Let me walk with you a minute," I suggest, and as we move toward the hall I explain my request: "She's also very sensitive about being talked about." Once around the corner from the group we pause and I ask her to elaborate.

"First of all," she explains, "I notice when Helen has a sudden change of behavior, such as getting up and walking with purpose. That means something. And she is very sensitive about her mastectomies, and about her body being exposed and observed. She's very modest. I respect that by, in dressing, for instance, helping her with her shirt or blouse from behind, rather than facing her. Taking time is very important and helpful, too. I don't rush. And I explain what I'm doing, or about to do. I ask permission."

She says again that she has no trouble with Mom in toileting. She just feels that it has to do with respecting her and giving her dignity. The words fall on my ears like blessings.

As we talk, Trish goes by, which doesn't seem to concern Mary, but after about ten minutes she tells me, "I need to stop. I don't want to be seen talking to you when the nurse comes in."

I return and visit with Mom a while longer, replaying the conversation in my head, recalling what Mary says Mom told her when they were finished in the bathroom: "I'm glad you were here."

Not more than I, Mary.

October 11 Sometimes I'm hopeful that something positive can come from this. That we'll not only get through this crisis but that from it will evolve an environment far better than before. Better for Mom, and all the residents; better for us; better for the staff.

October 12 I find my mother outside, sitting alone on a bench in the cool autumn sun. "I don't feel good," she tells me. Her face is puffy. Congestion rattles in her throat. Her legs are covered with rash up to the knee. Her feet are swollen.

"Do you think you should be outside, Mom? Maybe you'd be more comfortable indoors."

"No, I feel safer out here."

I discover that she has had diarrhea. Did she know or sense this, and retreat out here alone?

I go looking for help, and am glad to find Mary. She and I work together to clean Mom up. Mary is very calm, very good with Mom. I could learn from her. She tells Mom everything that is happening, what she is doing and why. Mom, too, is patient with this unpleasant task. She doesn't swat. Nothing like that. When we're finished, Mary thanks me for being there. I thank Mary. Mom thanks Mary. "That's what I like about Helen," Mary says. "She always says thank you."

I take Mom out to lunch. She looks and seems to feel much better. We have a good time at the restaurant and listening to Perry Como afterward in the car. But as soon as we're back and in her room she shoots me a long, penetrating look.

"I'll be back tomorrow," I promise.

"No. I'm not staying," she tells me. "It's like *West Side Story* here."

She gets up off the bed and goes to the window. She looks out for long seconds, her back to me.

She doesn't want to accept the fact that I am leaving, and that I am leaving her here. She has decided to leave me first. I go out quietly.

October 15   At this second special Staffing in a week, Betty makes an opening statement about the importance of communication, echoing her emphasis of seven days ago. The first topic on the agenda is toileting. Terry and I share our positive observations of Mary in her interactions with Mom—her alertness to behavioral cues, her careful patience, her respectful demeanor, her explaining to Mom what she's doing. "My mother doesn't swat at Mary," Terry says. "She doesn't fight her, she thanks her."

"So the toileting is all much better now, right?" Betty says.

"No, not really," Meg says. "Sometimes better, sometimes not."

Does Betty not grasp that our intention was to provide an example of a skilled and successful approach to the problem at hand? Is she blind to the notion that outcomes can be influenced by her staff?

Although Terry and I came to the meeting hoping to see Mom's thioridazine dosage reduced, the decision is to leave it unchanged. We don't press the issue. Given my ever-growing mistrust of the competence and even good will of the staff, I'm *afraid* to reduce it so close in advance of our schools trip later this month. I don't want to hear claims of even more problems when we're a thousand miles away.

Near the end of the meeting Betty says that it's necessary to weigh Mom's best interest against everybody else's best interest. "I don't see those interests as mutually exclusive," I say.

My hope is fading.

— 20 —

Everything is a grace.

—Thérèse of Lisieux

"I don't want to bite anybody."

—Helen

October 17, Year Three Terry's mother has fallen. The night nurse says her head is gashed and probably needs stitches.

I arrive at Holly Hills. My impression is that the head wound isn't too bad, but I think it's possible that she has broken her hip and I request an X-ray. While Mom lies in bed with her bruises and her head gash and her painful hip, a nurse comes in with her morning dose of thioridazine. I refuse it.

* * * * *

Wayne tells me that she was laughing and joking with the X-ray techs, and even ate a good breakfast, but when I arrive she is in pain and can't get comfortable. The doctor calls. The X-rays show a fractured hip. She needs surgery.

It's midday by the time I ride to the hospital in the ambulance with her. I have to think through the Do Not Resuscitate order again prior to surgery. It remains an unsettling question; all the more so in the very midst of this army of doctors and life-saving equipment. I call Sharon. We decide to continue with the DNR directive.

More diagnostics.

More waiting.

Suddenly the surgeon appears. He explains the partial hip replacement procedure to us, says that she'll be able to bear weight immediately, and so will start physical therapy tomorrow. At 7 p.m. they wheel her into surgery, Mom not knowing where she is going, Wayne and I not knowing when or whether she will return.

October 18 Mom is in quite a bit of pain. And with good reason, judging by the size of the zipper-like scar on her right hip that hides the titanium beneath. The effects of the anesthesia are still pronounced, but when she's awake she's not shy to smile. Except when the aides or nurses or the physical therapist do something that hurts her. Then she yells, "Wayne! Wayne! Stop that!" Is she blaming him, or asking him to make *them* stop?

When the nurse picks her up in a face-to-face "hug" to transfer her from bed to chair, the unfamiliar procedure scares Mom, I think. In an attempt to "hold on," she clamps her jaws around whatever is nearest, which happens to be the nurse's shoulder. "Don't bite. Don't bite," the nurse says gently.

"I don't want to bite anybody," Mom answers.

When they need to lay her down Wayne helps, supporting her shoulders and head from behind and reassuring her that he is there and that she is safe. Somebody picks up her legs and they pivot her, and as soon as she is lying flat on the bed she exclaims, "Thank you! Thank you! Thank you!" When the two nurses leave, she waves to them and calls out, "Thank you, girls!"

* * * * *

Although Terry and I have assumed, with decidedly mixed feelings, that her mother will return to Holly Hills after her discharge from the hospital, we are informed otherwise this afternoon during a brief visit to Mom's room by their social worker. "We have no appropriate bed for her," she says.

Seconds pass. Neither Terry, nor I, nor even Mom says a word. We just look at her. And then she leaves.

October 19 I stop by Holly Hills to pick up my mother-in-law's clothes. The two staff who were on duty when Mom fell are present. "How is she doing?" Tess asks. I tell about Mom's surgery, her pain, and that she now has no home.

I ask her to tell me about what happened two mornings ago. Tess says that Mom had hardly slept during the night and that she has had numerous such nights lately, poor or little sleep for weeks. She points to where Mom fell on the smooth vinyl tile, where she hit her head on or near a brass utility-access plate embedded in the floor.

"Did she trip on something?" I ask. "Run into some furniture?"

"No," she says. "She just fell. She was half asleep."

A male aide joins us. "We've been instructed not to talk to you about these matters," he says, directing his message as much to the two women as to me. He says that they are to refer us to Betty.

"Why is that?" I ask. He says he thinks it's so that we will not get conflicting versions. So that the information we receive is consistent.

"It's important to us to understand what happened," I say. "I've always believed that first-hand information is the best." He moves off without responding and my conversation with Tess and her colleague comes to an end as well.

The electric lock on the Unit door fastens behind me. My eye is drawn to the little sign in the drugstore frame that hangs on the wall to my right: "They are not residents in *our* facility, we work in *their* home." I've seen it before, italics and all. I wonder now what it means.

Dementia takes many things from a person. From my mother-in-law it has taken memory, home, much of language, more of security and independence, many friends. But it has not diminished her perception, her integrity, her wholeness. It has not taken *her*. Despite her physical and intellectual breakdown, in this dark hour she seems, paradoxically, brightened and enlarged.

As I step outside into the jolting autumn sunlight there comes a new thought, yet one which seems instantly a remembering of something I once knew: Dementia also brings things. Blessings.

— 21 —

When anger arises in the mind, when fear becomes present, it can either make life hell or reveal another opportunity to enter into heaven.

—Stephen Levine

The mind is its own place, and in itself
Can make a Heav'n of Hell, a Hell of Heav'n.

—John Milton,
"Paradise Lost"

October 22, Year Three   Terry and I have had to make hasty arrangements for Mom to live at another local nursing home, Meadowlark Health Care Center, and I ride with her now as she travels there from the hospital in the facility's van. Lying next to me, on the seat behind the driver, is some paperwork accompanying her transfer. It describes her as having "Alzheimer's, recently escalated to aggressive behavior." The writer adds, "Expect this to be a difficult behavioral management case. Will cover with Haldol as necessary."

Meet Helen. You might want to keep those antipsychotic tranquilizers handy.

I drop the packet on the seat, reach back to where she sits, stoic in her chair, and take her hand. "We're going to your new place, Mom," I tell her with forced enthusiasm. "We're going home."

The van bumps and sways, dropping me into a hypnotic trance . . .

In my mind's eye I see the vehicle from far above, snaking along the city streets. A window opens slightly and something peeks out—the transfer papers—fluttering and convulsing at the opening. Soon the sheets break free, first tumbling and twirling in the vehicle's slipstream, now whooshed upward by the chaotic eddies generated by the traffic behind. Rising, floating, they are caught by a breeze which sends them streaming ahead of the van, directly toward the sprawling building which is our destination.

Suddenly, by some friendly magic, the light of the sun bursts the pages into flame, quickly reducing them to a thousand tiny motes of ash. As our driver pulls into the lot and parks, the thinnest of clouds settles quietly to earth all around us. Invisible. Harmless.

October 26   Mom is housed with the general population here, as the Secure Unit is reserved only for residents with both the inclination and the ability to leave the premises.

The majority of the residents Terry and I have seen are non-ambulatory, some able to propel their wheelchairs by their own efforts, others chauffeured to and from the dining room three times each day by overworked aides who often guide them in tandem, one in each hand. Most of the residents appear to be afflicted with dementia of one kind or another. I find the atmosphere of the place depressing, dominated as it is by severe physical and mental sickness, hopelessness, and ever-present curses and moans.

The staff, from top to bottom of the hierarchy, are quite accepting of dementia and its attendant behavioral manifestations. An occasional flailing of arms or gnawing of a shoulder are viewed as entirely normal, to-be-expected behaviors. "That happens all the time," they tell us. "That's the way it is with dementia."

No behavior-modifying medications are currently prescribed for Mom, nor were they used at any time during her hospital stay. None have been suggested by the staff here.

Janet, the evening nurse, is trying to arrange Mom's legs in a better position in the bed. Something hurts and Mom swings out, connecting with Janet's jaw.

"That didn't hurt me," she says to Mom, ". . . much." It's a terrific dead-pan delivery. Later, she stops me in the hall. "Is that all the harder she hits?" she asks.

November 1 Mom walks about fifty feet today. Her strength and effort are good, although I find the actual mechanics of her motion surprisingly clumsy. As though walking has become for her a foreign, unnatural act.

Terry and I were told at the hospital that she would probably be walking within a week, but after two weeks we don't see anything like that happening. Mom herself doesn't seem too eager most days. Mitch, the physical therapist, says, "She walks when she wants to, and doesn't when she doesn't."

November 2 There has been no consistency in providing my mother the assistance she needs to use the toilet. The expectation of many of the staff is that she urinate and defecate in her diaper, which they inspect on a regular schedule and change as needed. Whether as a result of this, or as a consequence of her dementia—which seems to have deepened dramatically in the aftermath of her surgery—Mom less and less asks to go to the bathroom. More and more she fulfills their expectation.

November 3 My mother-in-law is withdrawn, aloof almost, since her fall. She sits in her wheelchair, tall and erect, gazing around, not saying a word. What does she *do* from morning to night? What's going on in her mind? How does she feel?

I seem to be wanting something from her. Today, as I look at her sitting there in her chair, it hits me: she looks like an old person in a nursing home. I want her not to.

November 5 Mom is wearing some sort of padded boot. Terry asks the aide about it and she says she thinks that Therapy has put it on her. But when I ask Mitch, he seems to know little about it. He thinks maybe Nursing has done it.

We learn from the nurse that Mom has a blister on her heel. She thinks it is the result of her walking her wheelchair—pulling herself along with her feet. I point out that when she walks the wheelchair she walks on her toes. Mitch agrees and thinks the blister probably developed in bed. Sure enough, we notice now that she bends her right leg, knee up, and nervously pumps it, rubbing the heel on the sheets. The result is this ugly, angry red sore.

No walking today.

November 6 "Everything's such a mess," Mom says to Wayne and me. She seems as discouraged as I.

Sometimes I wish that she could just die. Especially now, now that she can't walk, and that she's got this new bedsore problem going on. Who knows what that will lead to? I don't have much hope that my mother, who only wanted "to be a real old lady and be able to walk," will ever do so again.

Maybe the truth is that nobody wants to do the things that need to be done, or *can* do the things that need to be done, to make Mom's life better, or to get her walking. Not social workers, not therapists, not nursing homes, not us. Not even Mom. Maybe the *world* doesn't have the resources.

November 7 Terry and I wedge into Martine's tiny, windowless social worker office, joining her and several other staff members for the first Care Conference on Mom since her arrival two weeks ago. A heating system fan rumbles like a cement mixer behind my head as Mitch gives the Therapy report in his gentle whisper-voice. Six feet away, I am forced to lip-read in order to patch together his summary of therapy progress and plans.

Someone notes that agitation has been observed in Mom. This triggers an appearance of the Care Plan, along with its familiar, institutional structure: goals, methods, measurement. A goal and measurement are quickly defined—"We will have not more than two periods of agitation in a day." If there is a method, I've missed it.

Terry speaks about Mom's strengths: her sense of humor, her outgoing personality, her verbal and social skills. She has no official report to make, though, and has to find ways to work her ideas into the conversation. I suggest that when giving Mom instructions staff talk in short sentences and use simple vocabulary. "Go step by step," Terry adds. Martine jots these ideas down.

Renee, head nurse on Mom's hall, suggests another goal: "No skin breakdowns." Martine puts pen to paper, then pauses. She adjusts herself in the chair, reworks the grip on her pen. "Maybe we should re-word this," she says. Renee proposes a solution, quickly adopted: "No further skin breakdowns," Martine writes.

I see. If Mom's foot falls off tomorrow, the goal at the next Care Conference will be "No additional feet falling off."

It's reported that the blister on Mom's foot is worse this morning. She kicked her bootie off during the night and rubbed the welt into a larger, deeper, and more dangerous purple sore. Mitch suggests a different kind of boot, a better one. There is general agreement, but this will require a doctor's order. "I'll call," Renee volunteers.

I request a copy of Mom's medication listing so that we can review it for accuracy. Martine isn't sure if this is permissible. She refers me to the Medical Records office.

"What is your policy on toileting?" Terry asks. No one answers. Finally, Martine suggests we talk to the nursing staff. Renee says nothing.

As she promised, Renee called the doctor immediately after the meeting. But an hour and a half has passed with no response, during which time we have watched Mom rub her heel on the mattress without pause, kicking off the protective boot within seconds each time we replace it.

The ulcer interferes with Mom's walking therapy, and I believe it's a serious injury in its own right, so *I* call the doctor. This upsets Renee and causes tension between us, which causes tension between Terry and me—and in Mom, who senses the tension in all of us.

When she returns to her room after her shower, Mom and I rejoin the Battle Of The Boot, wherein I try everything I can think of to keep the little blue boot on her and she repeatedly, skillfully, kicks it off. Terry thinks it might help to get her into the wheelchair which, working together, we manage to accomplish. Mom grumps at me when I try to teach her how to use her hands on the wheels. She sticks her tongue out at Terry.

We take her into the dining room to eat; she pushes herself away from the table. I fight her a little, but finally conclude that she isn't so much trying to get away as to go somewhere else. When I back off, she immediately rolls up next to the activity director, who is playing the piano across the room. For ten minutes Mom sings and sways in time to the music.

She still has life in her. She's trying to keep control of that life as best she can. Could I do as well?

November 8 I stop in to see our friend Jeb at his music store. I tell him about all the things that have happened these past weeks. "Wayne and I feel so behind all the time," I say. "We can't catch up."

"Life is always one step ahead of our control," he tells me. I nod gloomily but Jeb's eyes brighten. "That's a good thing," he says. "That's how miracles happen."

November 14 Janet tells Wayne and me this evening, "She smiles from the beginning of my shift to the end."

November 15 A friend of Terry's and mine is dead. Suicide.

This evening, on a long, solitary walk under naked trees, I ruminate about Holly Hills Health Care. I've been angry for a long time, eager to blame and punish them for Mom's fall and everything leading to it.

Tonight, though, assigning blame doesn't seem so important. And even should I succeed in extracting some sort of retribution, what will I have accomplished? Will I not simply have damaged some individual or group? Damaged the world? Whatever the reason for her fall, and whoever, if anyone, may be responsible, Mom is who and where she is. Right now.

I don't know other people's hearts. I don't know the pain, misgivings, and sufferings of their lives. I didn't even know it about my friend.

November 16 Leona and another aide come in with their gear. "Hi, Helen," Leona says, moving close to my mother-in-law's bed, ear probe in hand. "Can I see if you have a temperature?"

"No," Mom tells her.

Leona pulls back slightly, but she is not deterred. "Can I just see what your temperature is?" she asks again.

"I don't have a temperature," Mom says.

"Well, can I just measure it and see what it is?"

"No." She says the word louder, enunciates more precisely—insofar as such a thing is possible with her simple message.

Leona moves in closer. It appears that she intends to get this temperature at all costs. I just sit here, off to the side, and say nothing. I want to see what will happen next.

Leona moves nearer still. She rests her hand on Mom's chest. "Could I just for a second? . . . I'll just take it for a second." She leans ever closer, guiding the thermometer toward its docking station.

Without further warning and with impressive speed and precision Mom slaps her hand away. "No!" she says.

"Well, you know, I'm . . ."

Four times Mom has answered, clearly and unambiguously. I'm nearly ready to slap Leona myself. "Could you try a little later?" I suggest.

"Well, they like us to do it now. The nurse wants us to do it now."

I swallow a sigh of exasperation. "Mom, would it be okay if Leona takes your temperature?"

"Okay," she says.

So Leona sticks the gadget in her ear, and Mom lets her. The reading is 97.1. This seems to be what her temperature always is with this thermometer. Leona does not question the results. She writes down the number on her form.

"You were right, Mom. You don't have a temperature!"

The other aide approaches, warily, with a blood pressure cuff. "May I take your BP?" she asks meekly.

"Yes," Mom says.

She slides the cuff up Mom's arm, secures it, pumps, listens for the pulse. Leona lingers at the foot of the bed, facing away from Mom and me. Mom catches my eye, then glances toward Leona, then back to me. She thins her lips and silently shakes her head.

"It's real good," the second aide tells Mom when the blood pressure is done. "143 over 74."

A moment later they are out the door.

"So tell me about that lady, Mom."

"She's taking my BP."

"Yeah, and what about the older lady?"

She shakes her head like before. "No," she says. It is not a refusal to tell. It is the telling.

"I understand that you didn't want your temperature taken. You said no very clearly. I think both you and I knew that you didn't have a temperature, and I really appreciate how patient you were with her." I pause, giving her time to digest, to respond. I see nothing outward, but her eyes are bright and I sense that she is with me. We are having a conversation. My part is just louder.

"I feel a little bit for her, because she's a nurse and her job is to take the temperatures." I give Mom a quick smile. "She doesn't know what to do when you say no. I wish that she could be different, but I don't know if she can. . . . They're trying to take care of you, and that's one of the ways they know how to do it."

Mom looks at me serenely. I do my best to mirror her calm.

November 17 Nudging the aluminum walker ahead of her, Mom lurches the length of her hall, past Terry and me, past the entry to

the dining room, and on toward new frontiers. Mitch, the physical
therapist, walks a half step to her side and behind. I don't think
Mom is aware of him, although his sturdy hand never loosens its grip
on the blue nylon safety belt that encircles her waist.

At the moment, he is not supporting her much. She is walking
more strongly than usual, although her right foot is very crooked,
pointing to the left at an angle of nearly forty-five degrees. The new
protective boot she wears on it is huge, shiny and hard and plastic,
like a ski boot. She keeps catching it, hooking it behind her left foot
with every attempted step. How can she not? It must be like walking
with a weighted swim fin on one foot. She has a natural ability,
though, and repeatedly frees it from entanglement as she plunges
on, veering steadily to the left, like a car in serious need of an alignment.

Now her foot catches badly. She staggers, and the walker skids
far out in front of her. As she pitches forward, the tendons in
Mitch's right forearm tighten and his left hand goes to her shoulder.
But for perhaps one toe in tenuous contact with the tile, Mom dangles for a moment in midair. "Oh, come on!" she exclaims in a tone
of impatience and annoyance, regains her balance, and plows on-
ward. Coming upon a soft and inviting chair she sits, panting, need-
ing the rest. But the chair is deep, and when she is ready to continue
she cannot get up. "I need a man!" she announces with enthusiastic
ambiguity.

"This is a good man right here," I suggest, pointing to Mitch.

She accepts his help and is up again, this time heading for Barney, a resident whose flannel shirts have marked him as her older
brother since her arrival here. She is animated and curious, looking
all around, even as she pursues her ersatz brother. Along her route,
her favorite staff member from Cottonwood Adult Day Care—now
a Meadowlark Health Care worker—suddenly exits the kitchen.
Mom recognizes him immediately, shoves the walker forward and
extends her right hand, maintaining a precarious grip on the walker
with her left.

"Hi!" she says with a grin.

November 18 My mother's engagement ring is gone. I report it to the social worker. She gives me a form to fill out.

November 20 I take my mother to her room after breakfast. Almost immediately an aide wheels her roommate Cora in. I play some Perry Como selections, show Cora Mom's picture of Perry, and tell her about Mom having been a singer.

Cora's eyes light up. "Oh, sing a song!" she says.

Mom and I sing "Pennies From Heaven" and "Temptation." Mom remembers all the words and delivers the songs with a strong voice and remarkable stage presence, looking Cora right in the eye as she sings. Cora, her hand possessed by tremors, leans toward us and manages to take hold of Mom's arm. "Thank you," she says as we conclude, then adds, "That's a wonderful picture of Perry Como."

Mom smiles sweetly at her. "You can't have it," she says.

November 22 Medicare covers thirty days of rehabilitation services after hospitalization, after which a decision is made about the likelihood of further progress and whether continuation of such services is warranted. Mom's thirty days are up. She is being taken off Medicare today and moved to a non-Medicare room. There will be no more physical therapy for walking. Wayne and I are giving up the hope that she will ever walk again.

But if they love her, if they can give her peace and stability and make her feel at home here, if she loves them, maybe it's not so important whether she's walking or rolling, maybe it's not so important whether she relieves herself in the toilet or in her pants. Maybe those things are not what it means to be a human being.

*Anybody who is familiar with nursing homes knows that there
are few things in that environment that really are under a person's control.*

— Jon Kabat-Zinn, Ph.D.

December 4, Year Three   I slip a new music tape into
my mother-in-law's player, stepping out of her line of sight for a
few moments to do so. She forgets that I am here, rolls out of the
room and heads down the corridor. To adventure.

Ten minutes later I've finished visiting with another resident
down the hall and am returning to Mom's room to get my coat as
she approaches from the opposite direction. Her eyes light when she
sees me and she reaches out with both arms as to a long-lost friend.
"Waaynnee!" she exclaims with utter amazement and unabashed
glee.

Infected with her joy, I throw my arms toward her.
"Moommm!"

December 7   I guess we haven't fully given up hope of Mom
walking again after all. Wayne offers her the walker, as much for
distraction as anything, and, to my surprise, she gives it a try. But
there is too much clutter and congestion: people crowding up behind in wheelchairs, others bearing down on her head-on, nurses
pushing bulky medicine carts, a young man mopping the floors,
visitors. She can't focus; she's constantly looking around to see
what's going on. All the while, we're moving her out of someone's
way, or moving them out of *her* way.

We give up and go to the TV room. A respite of sorts, until the staff start wheeling people in for lunch, which won't be served for over an hour. First comes a fellow who alternates between moaning and calling out in a deep, bellowing voice words that are completely unintelligible to me. I feel sorry for him, but I'm also angry at him for making these noises, for being so ill. He's doing the best he can, I tell myself, but the admonishment doesn't help.

Now comes a crying lady. As soon as the aide lets go of the wheelchair she starts rolling herself around. First she parks square in the doorway, blocking it, now crashes into a chair, and now *she* starts moaning. Mom looks in her direction and all I can think of is what she said in the hospital the first night she came to Colorado: "I can't get better here."

There's so much sickness everywhere—all this coughing and moaning and yelling—so much distress and agony that I just want to get away!

This is where my mother *lives*. Today, I can hardly bear to visit.

December 12 My mother is prone to urinary tract infections and we've noticed that they typically diminish her physical and mental functioning across the board. So when I noticed four days ago that she was having difficulty eating, drinking, and talking, and that she had mucus in her eyes, I requested that they do a urinalysis. Late the following day we learned that a UA had not been done. Urine was finally drawn last night.

This morning a crew is cleaning the floors on Mom's hall. Not just mopping, but heavy-duty cleaning—stripping old wax and applying new. There is a strong chemical smell in the whole area and we are alarmed to find Mom in her wheelchair out in the hall, sitting amongst stacked furniture and in the very midst of the fumes. She is in a stupor. We immediately take her up to the front door for some air.

But the fumes are too strong for our liking here, too. We want to get her out of the building altogether. It's a sunny day, and very mild. I check with both Abby, the director of nurses, and with

Renee about taking her out, and they are both supportive of the idea.

We bundle her up and take her to a nearby cafeteria for lunch. She seems interested in eating, but once the food is in her mouth she doesn't chew very much or swallow, and so consumes almost nothing. By the time we get back to Meadowlark she is slumped in her chair, her mouth is hanging open, and her eyes are wide and staring. "Is my mom getting any new medication?" I ask Renee. She says she is not, and after shift change I speak to Janet, who says the same. But Janet agrees that Mom looks bad, so much so that she wonders if she has had a stroke. She isn't able to eat any dinner, and when we get her to bed she rolls onto her side and falls quickly asleep.

At home Wayne and I go to bed, too, not knowing whether Mom will still be alive when we wake.

December 13 Six a.m. Mom looks no better than last evening. Terry has brought homemade chicken broth in a Thermos and spoons it onto her mother's eager tongue. She loves it. Even gets a little down. Ninety minutes later at the breakfast table she is again unable to swallow.

At lunch she is far worse. Any food placed in her mouth by the aide or by ourselves oozes back out, dribbling down her chin and neck. Her breathing is labored, though she sits motionless at the table. She leans hard against her seat back; her body is tensed and rigid, seems thinned, elongated, as though she is being suctioned from the chair by some unseen force in the ceiling above her.

Eye messages pass between Terry and me. It is clear to us, even as we continue our useless attempts to feed her—as though a spoonful of pureed potatoes might yet prove her salvation—that something is desperately wrong, that Mom might be dying, in silent, slow motion, before our eyes. It is a surreal scene, this private event unfolding in such a public place. I feel invaded by these dozens of people and the din and clatter of their usual business—eating, feeding, and being fed.

So little is being done. Nothing, really. No one seems to know anything to do, we among them. Perhaps there *is* nothing to be done. I feel as though Terry and Mom and I have slipped into some other dimension, that we are invisible perhaps, or have become a kind of specter, whose presence cannot be acknowledged by those who have another day to live.

Suddenly comes news: the urinalysis which Terry requested so many year-long days ago shows that Mom *does* have a urinary tract infection. But no sooner do we receive this information than the nurse tells us that she can't do anything. No medicine can be given without a doctor's order.

No. I understand that. But why then *isn't* there a doctor's order? What kind of health care system is this? She's dying! Can't they see that? It took five days to get a test done and have the results reported. Will it take another five to start treatment?

Calls are placed, but the doctor is in surgery or something. She can't be reached.

By 2 o'clock Mom is in dire shape. She is panting, her jaw slack and mouth open wide; her back is arched like a loaded bow, tilting her head so far back that she faces the ceiling. Her pulse is rapid, her blood pressure low. She can't talk, remains unable to eat, drink, or swallow.

A Complete Blood Count has been ordered, how or by whom we don't know. Maybe by Cynthia's efforts somehow. She's a nurse we have great confidence in, and she's been leaving helpful messages on our Voice Mail all morning, giving us updates and telling us where we can contact her after she goes off the floor at 2 p.m. Oddly, we haven't seen her, and she doesn't seem to know that we are here.

I learn that the CBC is not a priority (STAT) request, a circumstance that virtually assures me on this unlucky Friday afternoon that it will take days to get the results. Terry and I decide that Cynthia is our best hope and I ask at the nursing station to speak with her. Abby and one of the line nurses, Gina, casually discuss where she might be.

"She told me she'll be in the computer room," I tell them. Again they confer, in words I cannot distinguish. "I don't know where it is," I say, leaning over the high counter that separates us as though to speed my words to their ears. "She's out to lunch!" Abby snaps.

2:30. Still no call-back from Mom's doctor. Terry and I wait for thirty more agonizing minutes, keeping Mom company but powerless to provide relief. At 3 o'clock I call the doctor's office.

The receptionist has very little idea what is going on. She doesn't know who I am, doesn't understand why I'm calling for Mom. "Why doesn't *she* call?" she asks.

Somehow Cynthia has been found and joins us on the line at another phone with pertinent reports. I give way, relieved, but suddenly a testiness develops between her and the lady at the doctor's office, a skirmish about turf and chains of command and who has authority for what.

"As far as the CBC," I burst in—the two voices stop—"we're not asking the doctor. We're saying that if the CBC is important, then it needs to be ordered STAT. We want those results *now*. Tonight or tomorrow is going to be too late to do any good."

Ten minutes later Meadowlark receives orders for a CBC STAT and administration of Rocephin, an antibiotic. The shot is given. A technician arrives minutes later and draws blood.

Mom's doctor comes by in the early evening. She tells us it looks like pneumonia. "I don't know if she's going to make it through this," she cautions, and I wonder whether this is doctors' code for a harsher prognosis. Terry asks whether we should take her to the hospital.

"They'll just want to resuscitate her if she should die, and you don't want that."

"I don't," Terry says. "I just want to make sure she gets good care."

"She'll get the good care she needs here."

A moment passes before Terry speaks. "I don't know about that," she says.

Before leaving, the doctor orders IV fluids. It takes hours to arrange, finally gets set up about 10 p.m. After less than five minutes the apparatus malfunctions and shuts itself off. I tell Gina. She resets the device. Five minutes later it halts again.

Three times the identical scenario plays out. When the machine stops a fourth time, I read the directions on the unit, ascertain that the controller is mounted too low on the mast, adjust it upward a few inches, and restart it. After it runs continuously for fifteen minutes I go looking for Gina to tell her the good news and to explain the solution I have found. She seems pleased, but doesn't come into Mom's room.

At 11 o'clock, after a nebulizer treatment to soothe and medicate her respiratory tract, Mom falls asleep. Her IV is running smoothly. Terry and I leave for home. On our way we are stopped by the police. I have driven halfway across town with no headlights.

December 14 Terry's mother is weak this morning, but more alert. She reaches to stroke my cheek as I lean my head against the bedrail.

When breakfast arrives she immediately grabs the nearest item on the tray, a glass of juice, and tries to drink. She spills half of it, but she is involved and purposeful. She drinks, she chews, she swallows, she feeds herself. She takes her thyroid medication and nutritional supplements—three or four pills—without any instruction or assistance.

"How's the food, Mom?" It's a trite question, to be sure, but her animated reply—"Good!"—is not.

I have been told that she slept soundly last night and for that reason apparently did not have any nebulizer treatments after Terry and I left. We understand the order to be for treatments as often as every four hours if requested. When Mom finishes eating I ask Renee to give her one.

"Why?" she asks. "Why do you think she needs that?"

Her response feels aggressive. I don't understand why. Maybe it's me. Too tired. "Her doctor ordered it every four hours," I explain.

"It's PRN," Renee says.

"Yes. I know. And I'm asking for it."

Again she pushes for an explanation. My pulse rate kicks a notch upward. "The doctor ordered it," I tell her. "We think it's good for her. We want her to have it."

"Yes, sir! Yes, sir!" she says, snapping off her reply with everything but a salute as she goes to get the medication.

What's the choice? Just pick up and move Mom elsewhere, like changing rooms in a motel? If only it were that easy. There is no elsewhere.

Renee returns with the medicine. "I don't understand," she says as she loads up the nebulizer. "Why do you think she needs this? She's looking good to me."

"Yes, she is. That's why I want you to do it, I think it's helped. And the doctor ordered it."

"No," she says. "The doctor didn't."

She does not elaborate, does not show me the order, but I assume it is there, PRN—as needed or requested—as she herself said. Why else would she be readying the treatment?

She cautions that this medication is not something to be used in excess, that it is a strong bronchodilator. I tell her that I appreciate the information and that I respect her opinion, but that we want it for Mom at this time. "I don't want to argue with you," I say. "And I certainly don't want to argue with you in this place." Right over Mom in her bed, which is what we are doing.

The device is loaded with medication now, and Renee sticks the mask on Mom's face without warning or explanation, yanking the strap roughly over her head. Mom flails and knocks her hands away. I take the apparatus from Renee and place it myself, explaining my purpose to Mom as I do so. She resists at first, then calms as the vapors tumble into her lungs.

After lunch Renee comes in once more, this time to tell me that the doctor has written an order for a nebulizer treatment every six hours. "Whether she needs it or not," she adds in sing-song.

After shift-change I review some things with Janet—the status of the IV bag, the Rocephin and nebulizer treatments coming up. Our discussion goes quickly and easily. I leave just before three.

At six I return to feed Mom supper. She eats well, and drinks a lot of liquids. I ask Janet about the nebulizer. She says it went fine.

When I see her again at 7:30, feeling intrusive and pushy but driven to "make sure," I ask about Mom's four o'clock Rocephin dose. Janet says she didn't get it, that it didn't come with the IV.

My mind races. Does she mean it didn't come with the IV that was ordered and delivered nearly 24 hours ago? Is each dosage delivered separately? I remind her that just before I left at three she had said that she was going to give Mom the Rocephin shortly.

Janet leaves the room and I leave with her. Follow her around, asking questions. She unlocks the door to the medication room, slips inside, comes out empty-handed. She's on the phone. I hear her spell Mom's name. She goes again into the meds room, emerging this time with Rocephin. It was underneath someone else's similar or identical medication, she explains.

"Are you sure this is the right one?" I ask, as she readies the syringe in the hall outside Mom's door. "This isn't the other person's medicine, is it? This is the right medicine for Helen?"

"Yes, it is."

Her answer is without rancor, without defense. She enters Mom's room and installs the medicine quickly and effectively in the automated dispenser.

Just me and Mom now. Twenty-four hours ago she was near death. Now we've got a treatment started—it wasn't easy—we've got a little bit of a rebound . . .

Should I stay the night?

— 23 —

Anyone can respond with fear and anger. Our challenge is to respond with love.

—Marie Way

The only way to speak the truth is to speak lovingly.

—Henry David Thoreau

December 16, Year Three   This morning I find the door to my mother's room closed but for a few inches. As I near it I can hear screaming inside. I ease in, anxious and cautious, and find Delta, Mom's new roommate since the Medicare move, pulling at Mom's wheelchair and the oxygen tank attached on the rear. She is furious, yelling and making a racket, while Mom watches from her bed.

While I am deciding what to do, the speech pathologist comes in to assess Mom's eating ability and to see how she is doing generally. But we can hardly talk, can't hear each other over the yelling and banging. She goes and finds an aide who takes Delta out of the room. In the sudden quiet I am crying softly, telling the therapist about how I found Mom, and Delta, and the door.

Mom reaches out and pats my hair. "Don't do that, honey," she says. It's the most that I've heard her say in weeks.

December 17   The doctor told us yesterday that Mom's blood test last week showed that she was very dehydrated. Her electrolytes were completely out of balance and her kidneys almost failed.

There's always a pitcher of water by her bedside. But Mom isn't capable of using it. She can't reach it; doesn't even know it's there. This morning we've brought a sign to post by her bed, asking anyone who enters to offer her a drink of water.

But when Terry shows it to Abby she says that we can't put the sign up. Health Department regulations, she says. Confidentiality rules. I ask what regulation that might be so that I can speak to the Health Department about it. She laughs off my question. "They won't do anything," she says. "Patients have absolutely no rights."

Really? Even though she just told us that a primary reason for disallowing our sign is to protect Mom's right to privacy? Even though she has never objected to Mom's photo and biography which we posted on her door two months ago and which have been there for all to see ever since? Even though Mom, and we as her Attorneys-in-fact, can surely share any information about her she wishes?

"No, no, no," Abby says.

I ask once more about the regulation. She laughs again, and disappears down the hall.

Evening. Mom has been in bed for twenty minutes and is starting to nod off. I ask Gina about the possibility of her getting her meds before she falls asleep. "She's next," she tells me at the medicine cart.

Two minutes later she comes in with two medications—one of them discontinued yesterday, which I refuse—but not the medication I am most watching for.

"What about the new antibiotic?" I ask, knowing the injection order was replaced this afternoon with an oral medication.

"We don't have it in stock," she says. Her position on the matter is that they will wait until tomorrow to start the medicine.

"What about Meadowlark's 24-hour pharmacy?" I ask.

"It's so late now that it would be midnight or after before they would get here with it, and then we couldn't give Helen her 8 a.m. dosage."

Terry and I confer. I share our conclusion with Gina. "We think it's important that Mom get her medication as prescribed. We're not willing to wait until tomorrow. Or midnight, either."

"It was only ordered this afternoon."

"Why wasn't stock checked and the medicine ordered at that time? Maybe it'd be here by now."

A wall of tension divides us.

"Well, I don't know what to do," she says, hunching her shoulders.

"Well we need to do *something*. How about we get it from the hospital? I know you can't leave. You call it in, and I'll go get it."

"No. We can't do that," she says.

She does not explain why she "can't do that." Which is just as well, because I do not care why. I simply want my mother-in-law to receive the medicine which has been prescribed for her. I do not speak these thoughts. I do not speak at all. I do not even move.

Gina picks up the phone, dials, speaks briefly and quietly into the mouthpiece. I hear enough to guess that she has called Abby for instructions. She hangs up and I raise my eyebrows in question. "I'm waiting for a callback," she says.

"What does that mean? When will she call back?"

"I left the message on a machine."

"So there's no way of knowing when she will get the message, or when you will get a return call." She agrees. "Look," I say, "the administrator has told us that medications are to be given within thirty minutes of the prescribed time. It's now thirty minutes"—I glance at the clock—"make that thirty-*two* minutes past the prescribed time, and there's nothing in sight." I pause for a response but none comes. "We need to call him," I say.

She does so immediately and Mark tells her to get the drug from a local pharmacy. Moments later Abby calls and Gina tells her what Mark has instructed. She listens, nods, replaces the receiver. "She says not to do that," Gina explains. "She told me to have our pharmacist paged."

Gina carries out this new order from her immediate supervisor, even though it conflicts with that of the facility administrator. She hangs up the phone and we stare grimly at each other across the counter of the nursing station.

The pharmacist calls back within ninety seconds. Gina listens and, still on the phone, tells me, "They'll get it as soon as they can, but if you want it right away they could call it into Peterson's Pharmacy and you could pick it up. Are you willing to do that?"

"Yes."

Another two minutes and the phone rings again. The medication is ready at Peterson's.

I step out into the reviving December night air, drive the half mile, find Mom's medicine packaged and waiting, bring it back and hand it to Gina who administers Mom's first dose at 9 p.m.

Teamwork. Of a sort.

As Terry and I are putting on our coats to leave, Mom gazes dreamily up at her daughter.

"Kiss me," she requests. And Terry does.

December 18 Five hours after Terry and I left last night I return. Delta has been having a difficult time for days: calling out, screaming, rattling her bed bars, pulling on the curtain. I want to see how she is at night, whether Mom is getting good rest, and how the night shift handles things.

Mom is asleep. Delta appears to be asleep, too, though restless, and shortly after three she begins to mumble quietly, "Mama. Mama." Thomas, an aide, comes to the door, knocks lightly, goes over and says a few soothing words to her. She quiets again and he leaves.

At 4 a.m. Thomas again knocks and enters, this time for Mom, and I excuse myself. He pulls the privacy curtain and I hear him talking quietly to her, identifying himself and telling her that he is checking to see if she is dry, that he needs to turn on the light— everything he is doing.

"Oh, come on, goddammit! Don't do that," Mom suddenly complains. But in a few minutes Thomas is finished. I hear the soft rattle as he pulls the curtain open, and when he emerges from the room he is smiling as pleasantly as when he entered.

Janet brings Mom's antibiotic at 7 p.m. "I can bring it up to an hour early or an hour late," she says in what is apparently a pre-emptive strike. "I think it's better this way than waking her."

Mom has received her meds late three days out of the last four. We want to trust, need to if we're going to get through this. This is a step. "I think 7 p.m and 8 a.m. is very good for Mom's needs," I agree.

A step in a good direction.

December 19 As I am leaving this morning fear tightens Mom's eyes. "Don't forget me, Terry," she says.

"I never forget you, Mom."

* * * * *

Mom's meal is waiting for her when I roll her up to the table. She immediately spots the cake and reaches for it.

"She needs a good slap!" her tablemate exclaims.

I cringe inside, but respond light-heartedly. "Good evening, Melba."

"She eats like a pig!" Melba sneers in reply.

Again the words shatter against me. Mom shows no sign of having heard, but I cannot believe that they have no effect on her. She understands nothing, but understands everything.

Through the rest of the meal Melba is friendly and talkative. Mom? Not a word.

I wish it could be more pleasant, everything in the environment here. For Mom. For everyone.

Bless them all.

December 21 "Pretty fragile skin on her buttocks," Cynthia tells Terry and me after Mom's shower. She finds an extra piece of padding and places it on Mom's wheelchair seat. She also writes a note to the physical therapist about her skin condition.

But it's Saturday. Mitch won't be in for forty-eight hours, and the skin is fragile *now*. Isn't there something we could be doing before Monday?

I have a lot of mistrust. But I believe the energy that feeds it derives from a positive intention: that everyone here receive good care. Not only the residents, but the staff too, and the residents' friends, the residents' families. Everyone. My intent is to work together with this team for as long as Mom is here. How do I find the way?

* * * * *

Today is the Christmas party, but it's turning out to be a hard day. Wayne and I have been here since before lunch, but Mom just doesn't want to get up for the party. We give her her present from us, a Bing Crosby audiotape. It looks pitifully small and insufficient. Mom is more interested in the wrapping than the tape itself.

* * * * *

I catch sight of Norma, one of the therapists. She's done good things with Mom. I take her aside and briefly fill her in on the situation about Mom's skin as aides whiz past with residents in wheelchairs.

"I'm not working," she tells me. "I'm here for the Christmas party only." There's a protocol, she says. The protocol is that skin and wound care are nursing issues and must be initiated by Nursing.

"Cynthia has looked at Mom," I tell her, thinking this will fill the bill, but secretly longing for a time and place where skin and wound care might be considered patient issues as well, might even be initiated by *them*. "She's concerned. She left a note for Mitch, but since he isn't here and you are, and the two of you seem to work so closely together. . . . The aides will be changing her in a few minutes. I was hoping you could take a look and tell us whether a special cushion might be helpful."

"Here's the protocol," she says. "Don't inform me with your concerns. Inform Nursing. Nursing will inform Therapy. Besides, Therapy doesn't normally get involved until it's a stage two ulcer."

"What's that?"

"When the skin is actually broken."

* * * * *

After a short appearance at the party Mom is back in bed. "Terry, will you continue on . . . ?" she says, then loses her thought.

I think it would have been "continue on with me?" meaning that she wants me to stay. The truth is that I don't want to "continue on," not just now. It's 4:30. I've been here for five hours. I'm exhausted.

December 25 Mom has regained strength and abandons us frequently for self-propelled excursions down the always-new corridors. Today we find her in her chair, comfortably ensconced in the middle of the nursing station, surrounded by medical charts. I can almost picture her answering the phone and passing meds.

Later, as Wayne and I prepare to leave for other celebrations, I touch my forehead to my mom's, an intimate gesture that we have shared since her stay in the hospital two months ago. An expression of affection, and more: an homage, a blessing, each for the other.

January 1 We take Mom to eat at our dining hot spot these days, the cafeteria. She smiles at everybody who passes by, whether they acknowledge her or not.

"I was dreaming," she says in the midst of her meal.

January 4 Terry's dream:

Far off, a Zen Master sits in meditation. Her body becomes translucent. Her spirit gathers at her center and ascends through her chest, neck, and head, emerging above her body. Then a thought, as though infused: This is Mom. Mom is dying. . . .

This may be her time and way—this dementia, and even her fall—a way that she has created for herself to meditate, to "dream." Maybe she's dying and gaining a new experience of life at the same time. "I was dreaming," she told us the other day.

Wayne says he instinctively resists viewing her placidness in positive terms. But why? Why should we be less eager to put a positive light on it than a negative one? Is struggling to live the only honorable path?

Mom is going to die. Of something. Sometime. Is it not more important that her experience with us until that moment be one of love and peace than that we struggle to provide her an extra day—or ten years—of life?

All of life is sacred. This type of change, this passage through illness and debilitation, this is sacred, too. Dying is sacred.

January 5 Toothbrush in hand, my mother wheels across her tiny room, and in a sleight-of-hand maneuver that would make any magician proud, the toothbrush disappears. I search everywhere for five long minutes, finally find it, planted bristles up in the pot with Delta's poinsettia. Mom's engagement ring could be anywhere.

January 6 Cynthia calls. My mother-in-law has an open bedsore, one centimeter in diameter, just above her coccyx. Protocol, it seems, is satisfied.

Cynthia says she plans to treat the ulcer aggressively from a nursing standpoint. She's consulting with Norma for a better cushion for Mom, and has asked for a doctor's order for that. She says she will "put the screws on" the nursing staff to keep Mom cleaner and drier. The origins of the phrase depress me. Must the nursing staff be coerced through threat of torture to provide proper care? And if so, how about we keep those screws *always* in place? Mom's skin is fragile. No less so my loving resolve.

January 8   The ombudsman asks Mark if Cynthia might be promoted to Director of Nurses when Abby leaves in a few weeks.

"There's one problem with that," Mark says. "She's turned in her resignation."

This minute that comes to me over the past decillions,
There is no better than it and now.

—Walt Whitman,
"Song of Myself"

January 9, Year Three   I'd like to know what it's like inside my mother's head. What thoughts does she think when she wakes in the middle of the night? When I ask her what hurts and she doesn't answer? When she gazes serenely out the window? Is she resting when she goes into a reverie, or is she thinking active thoughts? Does she wonder when Wayne and I will come, or does she live in the moment, and simply see us when we're there?

January 12   A friend of ours comes with us today and brings his accordion. Wayne and I get popcorn for everybody while he sets up in the dining room, beams at the group, and belts out tunes. His name is Brennen but Mom calls him Courtney, after a boy in our neighborhood forty years ago whom he slightly resembles, and who also played accordion.

Brennen's is a new face and he brings the gift of music, but he is helpful in another, more basic way: just the very *fact* of his presence—that he is interested and willing to take the time—is uplifting. I return home feeling lighter.

January 14   The place seems to be falling apart. Aides and nurses keep disappearing—quitting or being fired. When I asked one of the staff recently about what remedies we might pursue for the kinks and twists and leanings that so mark my mother-in-law's posture of late, the reply I received was, "Maybe this is her 'true' position." Terry says there was only a single aide on duty on Mom's hall again. And despite Mom's need for it—and many others' as well—nobody puts out water anymore in the dining room.

Yet somehow, in the midst of all this disorganization, this institutional rush toward entropy, I feel the stirrings of something more positive. Something as yet unseen.

January 18   We've come to take Mom out to lunch. She's fresh from a shower but leaning in her chair like a haphazardly placed stack of books. Wayne and I struggle to straighten her, one on each side. As we lift, he under her shoulders and I at her knees, she leans toward him. He turns his face away and scrunches his shoulder, preparing to be nibbled. But gets kissed instead.

January 24   We arrive at 5:30 p.m. for the Soup Family Dinner. Quite a few families show up and the serving table soon overflows with bowls and pots and cauldrons of soup. Wayne and I keep busy with Mom and her tablemates, explaining the food choices and serving.

Martine, the social worker, tells jokes and reads poems. From time to time she invites others to share the microphone but there are no takers until Wayne volunteers. He reads "To A Mouse," a Robert Burns poem, complete with a heavy if imperfect Scottish burr. No sooner does he sit than a young man from the building maintenance crew gets up and sings "Food, Glorious Food!" from *Oliver!*

"Let's do the clambake song," Wayne whispers to me in a sudden competitive fever. He's talking about "A Real Nice Clambake" from *Carousel*. Not a bad choice, and we could probably do it. But I'm a little too shy. I was shy when *he* was performing.

Before he can muster a counter argument a thin, wavering voice rises from behind us. It's Bill, one of the residents, reciting a poem from memory. Something by Longfellow, I think. Bill gestures for emphasis with his one able arm and the words stream out, with much gusto but little volume, and only a handful nearby can hear him. Martine and Wayne contrive to get the mike to him just as he finishes, and it takes only a word of request to persuade him to launch into the verse again, from the top.

Everyone is connecting. Angie and her mom tell us a story from Angie's childhood; Marge introduces us to her mother, who lives on the Alzheimer's unit; I meet Claire, a member of the family support group, and her sister, a resident; Mark, the administrator, dressed in jeans, carries his darling little daughter, who becomes the instant focus of nearly every female resident who sees her. Gladys treats the baby as though it were her own grandchild, and when Melba can stand the wait no longer she calls out in an earthy, commanding voice that can be heard across the room, "Bring that little 'un over here!"

The entire scene is so far outside the normal turn of events here that the aides don't know what to do—but they're loving every chaotic minute.

A good thing is happening tonight.

February 2   Terry's dream:

Mom is talking on the phone to a friend. She's walking around. No chair, no walker, no limp. I'm surprised. And very happy.

I wake up feeling just the opposite: sad that Mom isn't walking, and almost surely never will.

But maybe Mom *is* having a good time, talking to friends and getting around as much as she wants to. Maybe she *is* doing well, and I constructed my dream to show myself as much. Maybe my mother is more in control than I know.

Wayne tells me today that he has been having a rapid-fire series of experiences and epiphanies about compassion and connection, that he's been seeing people and circumstances with what he calls his "soul eyes." He gives me an example. "I'm at the tire store yesterday," he says, "and the guy behind the chipped Formica counter is answering my questions about prices and ratings and warranties. I don't entirely trust what he's telling me; I can hear the salesman in him and I'm on guard. But then, suddenly—this has happened to me before—suddenly he transforms before my eyes. It's as though I see right past his skin to a person wholly new to me. An innocent, a being of flesh and blood and spirit who means me no harm, who's only trying to get by. To earn a living, to be successful at his work, to feel good about himself. Everyone in the store is the same, myself included. We are all the same—beings at once pitiful and glorious—trying to know ourselves and to do some worthwhile thing."

In some way that he says he cannot explain, he believes his experiences are related to Meadowlark and Mom and us. "I have the feeling that community could *happen* there," he says.

February 12   At Mom's Care Conference we learn that she has two open bedsores. A disturbing surprise. We thought they were healed for weeks. Wayne sees this as a potentially major crisis, one that could snowball out of control within hours or days. "We should have been looking at them ourselves," he mutters to me when the meeting adjourns.

"I love you," I tell my mom when I see her in the dining room after the meeting.

"Don't love me too much," she says.

"Why not?"

"I might not be here tomorrow."

February 16   When the nurse changes Mom's dressing today, Wayne observes her wounds for the first time. They are half an inch in diameter, one-eighth inch deep. Mom doesn't like any of the procedure. Removing the tape hurts, and she tries to swat the nurse's hand away. When this fails, she sticks out her tongue at Wayne. But as soon as the nurse is finished, Mom relaxes and smiles and seems completely comfortable.

I can't get myself to look at the wounds.

February 23 Eight inches of fresh snow on the ground this morning. We presume we will have to cancel our cafeteria lunch plans with Mom, but when we arrive at Meadowlark the parking lot is plowed and the sun is bright. We bundle her up in her coat, afghan over her lap, earmuffs, head scarf, and neck scarf over her mouth and nose. "I'm not cold," Mom's muffled voice assures us.

I've been learning about internet search engines and once we settle ourselves at a table I eagerly seize the opportunity to bring Mom and Terry up to date on the latest. "I don't understand any of that," Mom tells me when I pause for breath. "I don't either," Terry says. My audience is mocking me.

Mom gingerly reaches into the cranberry juice with her fork, fishes out an ice cube and delivers it to her mouth, then places the fork back in its cranberry "holder." When she drops a piece of chicken into a fold of her shirt she stabs it neatly. Just lowers her chin, squints her eyes, and impales it. And she does it all with as much aplomb and grace as if she is at a formal dinner party. Tonight's menu? Ice Cubes *Forchette* and Chest Chicken.

February 24 The standard introduction to Alzheimer's and dementia is that it never gets better, that there is no hope, that it only gets worse. We've been told this by professionals; we've heard it from families; we've read it in books. And, on one level, it's all come true. But I really do not see my mother-in-law's condition, or ours, as tragic. It certainly is difficult. It consumes great amounts of time and energy and effort. There are very poignant episodes which stick in my mind and probably always will.

And yet, despite all that, I have learned that when I live in the moment with her I experience wonderful times, times which are as good as any I have had with her—or with anyone—in my life. I look at her and smile, and she smiles back. When she has pain she flails at what she perceives to be its cause, but as soon as the pain stops she's not worried about it anymore. She's not complaining about it. She's not moaning about it. She's not fearing its return.

February 26   Wayne is at home, trying to drum up some book sales and school contracts. I've come to visit Mom but, as has become more and more the case lately, find myself involved with many of the other residents as well.

One of my favorite friends among the residents, Lucille, rolls her chair listlessly down the hallway, crying. "Hi," I say, and hug her. She tells me that she wants to see her mother, and all the relatives, and her dog, Peppy, too. Before I know it we're into a conversation about my dog and her dog, and how they're so much alike. She's laughing, I'm laughing.

I push Bessie in her chair down every hall three times over. "Take me where you're goin'!" she yells the entire time. I introduce myself to Wayne's friend Henry, and visit with Hilda, and Edie, and Henrietta.

Fascinating as they often are, I cannot long remember most of my conversations with the residents here. To do so would be like memorizing a very long string of unrelated phrases at first hearing. But communicating with the residents is not difficult at all. Communication with people who have dementia rides not so much on vocabulary and syntax as on tone and feeling.

"Nice girl! Nice girl!" Gertrude yells from her place at the table, as she always does when she is in need of assistance from one of the aides. Only it suddenly occurs to me now, after four months of hearing this same plaintive call nearly every time I'm here, that what she is saying is "*Nurse* girl! *Nurse* girl!"

Oh.

Make that tone and feeling and one's sense of hearing.

February 28   While Terry visits her mother, I attend a meeting with several other family members here who, like ourselves, actively advocate on their loved one's behalf, and who want to work with the staff to create a better environment for all who are connected with Meadowlark. We've christened our fledgling group the Family Council, and tonight we've invited the administrator to join us.

Mark comes in with a stack of forms which he spreads across the table. Some are six pages long, there are a dozen of them, and multiple copies of each. His idea is that we'll go through them, make comments and suggestions for improvements, then get together in a month to discuss. Oh my god, I'm on a committee.

But in the end I am feeling good about some of the values and goals Mark has shared. He wants to create a more homelike atmosphere here; he wants better staff/resident ratios. Just like us.

Who knows where this might go?

March 3   Wayne and I take Mom to Colorado Wound Treatment for her first appointment. She's been referred to this private clinic for treatment of her two bedsores.

Several CWT staff are directly involved with Mom from the moment she goes into the exam room: a nurse, a case manager, an aide, a physician. An impressive contrast to nursing home staffing patterns.

They take photographs of her wounds. The doctor comes in and debrides it—a procedure of cutting away necrotic tissue. In this instance, at least, it is a lengthy one and includes many painful painkilling injections. When the cutting is finished, they take measurements of the larger wound. It is 32mm—more than an inch and a quarter—in diameter. And it is deep.

As Wayne maneuvers Mom's chair through the doorway, the nurse reminds us of the importance of good hydration in the healing, and prevention, of ulcerous wounds such as these.

March 6   My mother-in-law is in bed, eyes wide. White, feathery hair frames her relaxed and glowing face. I put on Perry Como, leave, come back, repeat the cycle twice more. Checking on her, waiting for her eyes to close. "You look like an angel," I tell her.

"I know."

She says it without boast, and with another smile that only proves us right. I slip out, then in and out, in and out over the next half-hour; now tucking her teddy bear in next to her, now pulling the curtain a little to soften the hallway light on her face. I'm having fun.

Another few minutes and I peek in yet again from the doorway. I hear Mom's throaty voice, full of friendly consternation, but cannot make out her words. I move close to the bed. "What did you say?" I whisper, almost certain that she will not remember.

"I can't get rid of you," she says.

— 25 —

*Raising your love level is the only action that results in a
real change for the better.*

　　　　　　　　　　　　　　　　—Thaddeus Golas

"Go and love her. That's what they all want."

　　　　　　　　　　　　　　　　　　—Lucille

March 18, Year Three　As soon as the wound is un-
covered at Colorado Wound Treatment, my impression is that it is
worse than when I last saw it two weeks ago. The look on the physician's face, even before he speaks, confirms my suspicion.

"Has the wound been kept clean and dry?" The words spring
from his mouth like barbed hooks. It is a question neither Terry nor
I can answer.

More necrosis and undermining have occurred and, though he
does his best, the doctor is not able to remove it all. He suggests that
surgery may be needed and I think briefly that he is about to remove
Mom to surgery immediately. He clarifies that he is talking about
plastic surgery, that the wound is almost to the bone and might
require special reparative procedures, including reconstructive
surgery. He talks about possible admission to the hospital, maybe a
lengthy stay.

From time to time over the past thirty months, people have
suggested to both Terry and me that we are not accepting the reality
of Mom's condition, that we are in denial. I don't agree.

I don't think I'm experiencing anything other than a normal
grieving process over Mom's losses of ability or her eventual death.

What I do struggle with—and right now is a good example—is not grief, but anger. Anger about our culture's response to the dying process. Our denial of and fear of death demands that we prolong life, and the medical science community responds with ever more stunning and successful interventions. The interventions we supply, but the aftercare they necessitate—care which itself may be too remindful of death—we largely do not.

And so, Mom's successful hip surgery has not led to walking, perhaps because the best place she might have learned to walk again was in her own home. And although the government supports with its funding an isolating and segregating institution called a nursing home to accomplish that goal, the nursing home does not, perhaps cannot, do so. Instead, a bedsore develops on her heel and interferes with rehabilitation. Others, serious enough to require intensive intervention, develop on her buttocks and worsen to the point that reconstructive surgery and hospitalization may be required. Because of these ulcers she is necessarily less active, even somewhat bedbound, and pneumonia becomes a recurrent threat. Repeated courses of antibiotics fight the infections but encourage diarrhea and dehydration, both of which may interfere with, among other things, the healing of bedsores.

On and on, putting out fires, no doubt even igniting them at times, without ever looking at the larger picture. That we are willing to keep people alive but are unwilling to commit the resources to care for those extended lives, *that's* what makes me angry.

March 19   Terry and I sit at the table, finished with our dinner, our plates half-filled with uneaten food. "We need a new attitude toward the staff at Meadowlark," she says suddenly. "They're not doing a perfect job, but—"

"Oh, really? Gee, I hadn't noticed."

"Look, it makes me angry, too, when they screw up. But guess what? It's not going to work to always confront and browbeat them. It doesn't work for *me*. It makes me feel terrible."

"I don't think we browbeat them. We're looking out for your mom. If I could trust them to do what it takes to—"

"That's just it," she says. "I'm not talking about figuring out whether somebody's trustworthy or not. I'm talking about adopting a totally different attitude. I want to have an experience of beauty, and dignity, and compassion when I enter that building. Not just for the residents, and not just for me. For everybody. And if that's what I want, then that's what I have to bring. We get angry when we think the staff aren't carrying out their responsibilities. But how can anyone keep up her best effort without a feeling that she's creating something beautiful, without some acknowledgment of that from outside herself?"

"But haven't we tried that?" I say.

"Well, if we have, we haven't tried hard enough. It's the only way I can continue. Otherwise my life is choked with hate and distrust and confrontation, everybody at each other's throats. I want my Mom to *die* I'm so tired of it."

"We tried to build community at Holly Hills. Maybe we came in here a little on guard after that experience, but I don't think we've been unfair. Should we just keep turning the other cheek?"

"I'm not talking about turning the other cheek."

"What are you talking about then?"

"I'm talking about love. I'm talking about attitude. That's all I can say. I don't want to argue. Stay with the old way if you want, but I'm not going to do it. I *can't* do it. If a new way doesn't work, at least I'll have tried. If it fails, I won't be ashamed at least. I'll have done my best, what I believe in. The outcome isn't what's important."

"I know, I know. It's the process." I speak this final word like it's something foul. I'm not in the mood for ideals. "Well, what about this process of carving off little hunks of your mom one at a time? That's what niceness *leads* to." Wrong words, at a wrong time.

"We don't know why she has those sores," Terry says.

"Well I don't think it's because of the exquisite care she's gotten!"

"I'm not saying we can't do things about it, Wayne. But we've got to be compa—"

"No, wait. Tell me. What do we do after we've tried compassion, and dignity, and they just keep—her ulcers aren't being kept clean and dry, Ter! The doctor as good as said it. What do we do? Tell me."

"We deal with it! Okay? We deal with it. But going in angry and vindictive all the time is not—"

"I didn't start out that way. It's grown into that. It's like . . . like they've demanded it."

I'm not thinking straight. I agree with everything Terry's been saying, but all I can seem to do is fight. I take a breath, try a softer tone. "When you were talking about compassion, for everybody, it resonated in me. It made my heart lift up!"

"Really. Could have fooled me." *Touché.*

"It's not like it's a new idea to me, you know, or a new experience. I've had it hundreds of times in my life. And I love it when I do, because for that minute or hour or day everything is in harmony. I see beauty that in every other moment I can only try to convince myself that I remember.

"I had it for a while at Holly Hills, even after the troubles started. I went into those meetings with . . . it was really in my heart."

"Are you sure?" Terry asks. Her tone has softened, too.

"What do you mean?"

"Maybe it was just superficially in your heart, and—"

"And when people didn't respond the way I wanted I gave it all up and got cynical?"

"Something like that."

". . . Maybe so. . . . Maybe that's what's wrong with idealism. Mine, at least." She tilts her head in question. "That it's not true idealism," I explain. "As soon as I run into an obstacle I say, 'The hell with it.'

"I know you're right, about the compassion and everything," I tell her. "I'm angry because I can't find it within myself to do those things. One blow and I want to hit back." I take a breath, exhale hard before going on. "It was a mean thing, Ter, what I said about them carving hunks off of Mom. I said it because I don't like that it's happening. I wanted us to be mad together." I watch for some sign that my excuse-making apology has found its mark, but I cannot read her. "I'll tell you what I don't like about your 'new way' idea. It comes down to my having to be a saint, as though that's the only way the world can work."

"Maybe that is the only way the world can work."

"Yeah, well I don't want to be a saint. Let somebody else do it."

"Not just you. All of us."

Her words remind me of something Gandhi said, that we have to be the change we want to see in the world, and I give her a nod of grudging agreement. I can see that something more is building in her. And now it comes: "And you're also right that it was mean of you to talk about cutting off pieces of my mom. That really hurt!"

"I know," I say. "I know it did. But . . . it's the truth of it."

"No. It isn't. Don't you see?" She is angry, and pleading too. "We don't know the truth of it. We don't know why it's happening. We don't."

"I know it hurt you for me to say that, but it hurts me for it to be happening. I feel guilty about it."

"About what?"

"Everything! About all this stuff that goes wrong!"

"You're not guilty of it! Wayne, you have done so much for her."

"But she keeps getting worse."

"Because she's dying. We know that. But it's not important whether she dies a little sooner or a little later. What's important is that she die with as much love, and with as much grace and dignity, as she and we can muster. The other day Lucille told me, 'Go and love her. That's what they all want.' And I'm saying that not only should we love Mom and Lucille and the other residents, but all the people there, and ourselves too. We all deserve love, and dignity, and compassion. Just for being human beings."

26

"Be happy that we're all still alive."

—Lucille

April 17, Year Three   The last few weeks have been a continuing roller coaster, although the valleys have been less steep.

In late March, Liz, a nurse from CWT, tended to my mother-in-law's wounds at Meadowlark. It was a house call, nothing less.

The new director of nurses arranged for purchase of a special mattress for Mom's bed, a pneumatic device with computerized sensors and air delivery system to more constantly provide pressure relief to whatever body area needs it most. Both a therapeutic and preventative intervention. She even got the delivery date advanced so that the bed arrived in early April.

And the occupational therapist installed a new-and-improved seat cushion on Mom's wheelchair, as per doctor's order.

In the midst of such positive turns, Terry and I decided in late March—following a fourth consecutive meal at which Mom and many other residents were not served water—to undertake an active campaign to assure that every resident receives water at every meal. Our observations came on the heels of Mark's informing the Family Council that his staff was "studying the hydration situation" and that one method they had chosen to improve it was to serve water at all meals. A reasonable plan and a laudable goal, though in late March of this year, unattained.

Terry and I spent Easter Sunday with Mom, and soon after departed for a short school tour we'd managed to arrange in the Midwest, with friends volunteering to visit Mom while we were gone. When we returned on April 9, we told her what we'd accomplished and the places we'd gone; told her, too, that we were "back now" and think we saw sparks of genuine comprehension in her eyes.

On the evening of April 10, the director of nurses called us at home. She said the sore on Mom's left buttock was much better, the larger one on the right at least a little improved. She told us that Liz had been over not just once but a total of three times, and that no debridement was done or needed in her judgment. We kept bracing ourselves for the bad news. None came.

During Mom's appointment at CWT today the news is even better. As soon as they remove the bandage I can see that the large wound is improved. Still bad, but better. At its worst it was 1½ inches deep, now it is about 1¼. Undermining is still present, but the main thing is the tissue itself: pink and showing lots of granulation, it is immeasurably healthier looking. The doctor concurs and decides there is no need to poke or prod. We feel lifted in a way that we haven't before in connection with these sores.

"You're doing great," Terry tells her mother. "Your body's healing. It's doing a great job."

April 24   Wayne and I stuff envelopes for a Family Council mailing, using Mom's bed as a work table as she watches. Suddenly she speaks.

"Just promise . . . just promise . . ." She is looking directly at Wayne. Her tone is urgent, but she can go no further.

"Just promise what?" he asks.

"That you love me."

Her words, as well as an element of romance and passion in her voice, startle me. Has she mistaken Wayne for my long-dead father?

Maybe, but maybe not. Perhaps her request is nothing more than elementary, one that each of us makes, if less plainly, every day.

"I promise that I love you," Wayne tells her.

As we leave the building later, Lucille sends me off with simple, sage advice. "Just go home," she says, "and be happy that we're all still alive."

May 5   Although it seems to me that my mother-in-law's overall health has been slowly declining over the past months—one of my primary measuring sticks is her skill in eating and drinking—her sores continue to heal and she remains interested in everyone and everything around her.

She is one of the most placid people I've ever seen. And in the best sense. Always ready, able, and willing to smile, often enigmatically. She's like a queen, sitting there, smiling on her subjects. And not in a condescending way. More like she's blessing us. Like a great and loving laugh, though not a sound comes from her.

Mother's Day   Barney presents my mother a small bouquet. I don't know where he got it. She is smiling, pleased to receive flowers from her "brother." Brother's Day.

May 15   At CWT the staff do their usual photos and measuring, but already I have seen a look on Liz's face that does not bode well. When the doctor comes in he is strongly critical of the nursing care Terry's mother has received, which has allowed the healing wound to nearly close at the surface, even though tunneling still exists beneath.

But now he abruptly changes his tune, declaring that her comfort is the main thing. "We treat the person not the wound," he says and reminds us of something he told us early on, that we "should never expect this wound to heal." He advises that we maintain the wound as is, changing dressings daily for the rest of Mom's life.

But aren't premature closing and undermining problems? After ten weeks of progress are we to just give up?

A palpable tension pervades the room. Terry tries to elicit Liz's opinion, but Liz doesn't give it. In a matter of seconds communication has all but shut down.

"I feel like I have to make a decision right now," Terry says, "which I can't do."

"Can we have a few minutes to think it over?" I ask.

"Okay," the doctor says. "Take a few minutes." He reiterates his opinion on the issue, then adds, "If you want me to reopen it you'll have to make another appointment."

"When would that be?" I ask, uncertain whether the sudden frost in my heart chills my voice as well.

"Whenever my next appointment would be," he says, and leaves the room.

Liz remains. Terry and I acknowledge her difficult position, but ask her again what she thinks.

"I'll tell you what I think," she says. "I think you should get a second opinion."

We agree and Liz goes to check on possible arrangements. Within minutes she has secured an appointment for Mom with Dr. Barnes, the CWT Director, for the 19th, only four days hence.

The nurses place Mom in the mechanical lift, a sort of sling, which they use to transfer her safely from the exam table to her chair. Mom has been through this at each visit—suspended in the sling as it moves sideways, down, and rotates her simultaneously—but this time she panics. With amazing swiftness, her arm swings out in a wide arc and strikes one of the nurses on the head. Like human Velcro, her fingers latch onto a lock of the woman's hair.

I gently pry Mom's hand open, we complete the transfer, and soon she sits secure in the chair. "How's that?" Mom's recent captive asks with no trace of blame or bitterness.

"Fine," she replies, with an easy-going air.

And she *is* fine, her moment of panic long since forgotten.

27

*Problems cannot be solved at the same level of
awareness that created them.*

—Albert Einstein
(Attributed)

May 19, Year Three   Dr. Barnes is very cordial and
communicative with us. He decides to open the wound a little. The
appointment goes quickly and with little discomfort for Mom.
We're happy that he will be Mom's new CWT physician.

May 23   For two hours this evening I've been in the building,
dividing my time between Family Council business, visiting my
mother-in-law, and visiting with other residents.

I really like this. It's as though we're at home again, only it's a
bigger house, with more rooms and more people living here. And
even though I come from outside, it doesn't feel as though I'm a
visitor, but almost as though I live here, too. I can drop by at any
time of day or night, without calling, without an appointment, stay
as long as I want. I don't even need a key.

I feel like I'm a useable strand of thread that has been picked up
by some unseen cosmic tailor and put to good use in a garment that
is larger than I can see. We are all of us conscious threads and snip-
pets of brightly colored cloth. And all of us tailors, too, weaving
ourselves, instinctively and with the highest hopes, into the fabric of
each other's lives.

Mom's room. The middle of the night. Thomas, the night aide,
starts on his rounds. I whisper hello and he returns the greeting, an

inner glow brightening his eyes even in this dusky light. He remembers our December encounter, tells me it was exciting to him because he rarely gets to meet a family member.

When I come out of Mom's room a woman I do not know startles at my appearance. "Can I help you?" she asks, her voice cool and just this side of accusatory. I introduce myself. She tells me she is Lilith, the night nurse, and now she turns almost apologetic.

No need. She is protecting someone I love.

May 28   At the Care Conference, my mother-in-law's weight is an issue of lively debate. No one seems to know what it is, with reports ranging from 104 to 113 pounds.

She weighed 140 when she came to live with us, then promptly gained five pounds. Three years later her body has shed fat and muscle, like an ancient tree that drops its leaves in a final autumn. As though she understands that there is no need to bolster her strength but only to husband it. That before much longer she will require no body at all.

June 5   As part of the hydration program we first heard mention of more than two months ago, the staff started putting water flasks on the tables the day before yesterday. This evening I watch Terry's mother fill the drinking glasses for two people at her table. She doesn't spill a drop.

Not only hydration, but courtesies and graceful social interaction, too. All for the price of a flask of water.

June 8   My sister Sharon calls. They're thinking about driving out to Colorado, visiting Mom and spending some time at a small mountain resort. It's not only a visit, but a vacation, too. Sharon says she needs one.

So do I.

June 9   My strangest thought of the past day: I have to keep my mom alive until my sister arrives.

June 19   Wayne tells me that the director of nurses, the director of staff development, and the head of the Alzheimer's unit—nearly a quarter of the administrative staff—are quitting. I feel out of control. Scared.

June 28   Margaret is a new resident two doors down the hall from my mother. She is a smiling, friendly woman who talks freely about having Alzheimer's. She says that sometimes she wakes up and doesn't know her own name. "I used to be a nurse," she says. "Now I'm on the other end."

June 29   Since the 20th of June, when the nutritionist, Mindy, told us that she thinks Mom should be moved to a feeding table, Wayne and I have been watching Mom eat—when don't we? We can't see that she needs a feeding table, but yesterday she was moved.

There is no water at the feeding table. There is no room for me to sit next to her. So I watch from a distance. Although she is feeding herself quite adequately, a newer aide, Mallory, tries to get her to drink from a glass of milk. Mallory brings the milk toward Mom and Mom skillfully braces her spoon on Mallory's arm, deflecting it and its cargo. The scene replays. The third time, Mallory pushes Mom's defending arm to the side and gets the milk to her mouth. Mom leans back as far as she is able. Mallory tilts the glass. Perhaps a drop or two passes her lips.

Prior to her illness I never saw my mother drink milk. She told me that a doctor said that she's allergic to it. Although Mallory is sweet and gentle with Mom, I worry about ten different people forcing things on her that she doesn't want. Her quality of life during meals, one of the main activities of her day, is more important to me than weight gain or loss. I want meals to be enjoyable for her.

And I want to be able to sit with her at her table.

June 30   I am struck by how small my mother-in-law is, how little and flat and receded into the bed.

I find a red spot on her left hip and ask the nurse, Ryan, to look. He is aware of it, has been treating it. "It's looking much better than a few days ago," he says.

Good. I'm glad he's on top of it. "Do they turn her at night?" I ask.

"I can't speak for the night shift," he says.

No. I understand, but my confident appreciation of a moment ago crumbles to dust. His reply conveys such a feeling of disconnectedness among the staff that I can't relax. It forces me to live from shift to shift.

July 1   I feel so out of control. That's how I've been feeling for more than a year, ever since my mother left our house for California. I don't know what decisions to make sometimes, or what to even *worry* about. We could spend all our time dealing with Mindy and this feeding table, and it might turn out that a bedsore will kill her. Or we could spend all our time on bedsores and find out that she's hit in the eye by silverware thrown by another resident. She might fall out of her chair or bed. Or some other thing, something that hasn't even occurred to us, might be much more important. I don't know where to put my time and energy.

July 2   "How was your breakfast, Mom?"

"Not any more," she says with a smile, entirely pleased.

I fetch her some water as there is none on the table. I talk to an aide about our main feeding concerns—water, no milk, no forcing. Judging by her response, this is entirely new information for her. She is receptive. Gleeful, really.

At home, a phone call from the nurse Renee informs Terry and me that last night a staff person found a male resident in Mom's bed, with Mom. He was heard to say to her, "Hi, honey. What's your name?"

The man was removed from her bed.

Apparently she is none the worse for this incident, but it opens up a whole new realm of things to worry about that hadn't really occurred to us before.

July 15 My mother is enjoying eating outside! She plays with a little visiting dog, listens to the birds, and watches them eat from the feeder. She doesn't want to go in, even after the arrival of ravenous mosquitoes.

The meal itself is another story. It consists of a tiny glob of pureed tuna salad—which I sample and find to taste like the soggy cardboard it resembles—a little applesauce, Jell-O, and some juice. That's all. It looks like a child's portion. An appetizer. And Mindy wants her to gain weight!

She eats all of her cardboard tuna and applesauce. Plus three big cookies I've brought with me. Plus drinks a glass of water that Wayne gets for her. Plus eight ounces of protein shake that I have brought from home. Plus a serving of peaches that Wayne gets from the kitchen.

July 16 Mark tells the Family Council tonight that we're "just complaining." When a group member asks what the Family Council can do that would help him, Mark urges, "Do PR." He says that a higher census will bring in more money and allow him to hire more staff.

I don't get it. We want more help for the people who are already *here*.

July 17 My mother sits erect, smiling and looking downright healthy. And she has water at her table place! She grabs my hand and holds it, rubs my arm as though examining it, shaping it. My masseuse, my sculptor.

"Your fingers are dead," she tells me.

A few evenings ago she said to me, "I'm recalled." I couldn't figure out, then or now, what she meant. Now this morning my fingers are dead.

"Mom, you said my fingers are dead. You didn't mean to say that, did you?"

"No."

I believe her—that she tried to find the words, the ones to convey her real meaning, but couldn't. I think that's part of the reason why she's mostly stopped talking. It bothers her not to know how to say something. All her life she's been so articulate.

* * * * *

I run into Mindy just outside the kitchen and tell her about our preference that Terry's mom not be given milk with her meals, that we think it might be contributing to recurrent phlegm and mucus problems that she's been having.

Mindy tenses, positions her rotund body close and square in front of me. She says she feels very strongly that she wants Mom to have milk. She cites "her condition," and tells me, "I saw her, myself, pick up and drink unassisted an entire 180cc of milk."

I am surprised at the intensity of her response, but decide not to fight this battle right now; decide not to ask what my mother-in-law is supposed to do if she's thirsty and has no other choice at hand; decide not to tell Mindy that I've seen Mom pick up *flowers* and put them in her mouth. Unassisted.

I turn the conversation to another important—and surely less contentious—subject: the importance of water in Mom's diet, and our desire that it be available to her at every meal.

Mindy's response is to tell me "how difficult it is to get water to these people." She says this is for "various reasons," which she does not list. "This is extremely difficult," she says. "I'd have to make out a big long instruction sheet and do in-service with my staff." Which she agrees to do—on Monday.

"I want Helen to have water with her meals over the weekend," I say.

Mindy tells me that she works hard, seventy hours a week she says, and is looking forward to having the weekend off. I tell her that

I don't think Mom should have to wait. "Helen will have water at her meals this weekend," Mindy finally promises.

Although I don't agree with Mindy on the milk issue I can chalk it up to a difference of opinion and give her credit for good intent. But I simply don't understand how seventy hours doesn't result in a glass of water on every tray at every meal.

How *does* one ask for change, I wonder on my way to the car; how *does* one ask for a drink of water without being accused of complaining?

28

*A human life has seasons much as the earth has seasons,
each time with its own particular beauty and power. And gift.*
—Rachel Naomi Remen, M.D.

July 21, Year Three   The aide, Josie, feeds my mother-in-law breakfast. I see orange juice at her place, and milk. But no water. I get some for her and she immediately takes a drink.

I like the presence Josie brings to the table. She's very affectionate, reaching out to hold hands or sing as she performs her mundane assists. Mom watches her with a Mona Lisa smile.

"Does Mom feed herself?" I ask.

"Sometimes. Not always."

I notice that her plate is pulled about eight inches toward Josie. I surreptitiously slip it back toward Mom and, after accepting a few forkfuls from me, she picks up the spoon and starts eating eggs and drinking water under her own steam.

"I'd like some," Mom's tablemate says as she watches Mom drink.

"Some what?" I ask. You never know.

"Straight water."

I return with a glassful, and she quickly downs three-quarters of it in two big draughts.

"Thank you," she says.

After breakfast I spot Jody, a volunteer, with her dog and invite them into Mom's room. Chester is puppy playful and Mom lights up at the sight of him.

"Do you want to pet him, Helen?" Jody asks.

"Yes," she says and reaches out. Jody lifts Chester's paws onto her leg, Mom pets, and Chester sniffs and licks her fingers in a frenzy. "Oh my God!" Mom exclaims, with what sounds like equal parts fear and joy. This only inspires Chester to greater heights. He crawls his front paws up her chest, his long, pink tongue reaching for her chin. "Ohh!" Mom says—again part moan, part thrill—"Come on now."

After Chester's departure Mom brushes her teeth. I find her recording of "Just Out Of Reach" and put it on the turntable. Her grin shows right through the brushing.

"Remember that one?" I ask.

"Yrghhhhrhsgh."

I thought so.

* * * * *

My sister, her husband Denny, and their grandson have arrived from California. David presents his great-grandma with a new teddy bear—one identical to his present to her nearly a year ago—which she hugs and cuddles happily. The first has had a lot of loving wear and tear, but already it's obvious that Mom won't part with it. She's thrilled with twins. A trip through the laundry will have to suffice.

"How are you feeling?" I ask her at the picnic lunch out back.

"I feel nice."

Her face turns crimson, scrunches with emotion. She watches David intently: David juggling, David climbing the big maple, David jumping to the ground.

After lunch Sharon spends time alone with Mom in her room, her arm around her. After Sharon says her goodbye and leaves, I go in. "Have sweet dreams, Mom," I tell her.

"Yes," she says.

I believe she will.

July 23 Josie invites my mother-in-law and me to join her across the dining room in singing "Happy Birthday" to Hazel, who is 100 years old today. We sing, and Hazel thanks us all.

"Tell us, Hazel, what's the most important thing you've learned in a hundred years?" Josie asks in her best anchor woman style. She makes her hand into a fist, her thumb protruding like the head of a microphone, and places it in front of Hazel. White-haired Hazel doesn't respond immediately, the small knot of admirers before her as distracting, perhaps, as a rowdy crowd of reporters. Then the old woman reaches out, the skin of her hand like translucent porcelain, takes hold of the microphone-hand and starts trying to pry it open, unabashedly curious and determined to see just what Josie's hiding in there.

Immediately Josie shows her empty palm, then takes Hazel's searching hand in an affectionate grasp. "What have you learned in a hundred years, Hazel?" she asks again, this time without affectation.

"To . . . love everybody," Hazel announces.

We all clap, and Josie launches into a politically incorrect but absolutely celebratory solo of "The Old Grey Mare." When she is finished she tucks Hazel's chair back into its place at the table, releasing the guest of honor to her oatmeal and the start of her second century.

July 25 "This might heal yet!" Dr. Barnes enthuses when he sees that Mom's bedsore is doing better. We and the CWT staff shower each other with compliments. The doctor calls Wayne and me "troupers," and says that we are "real good at taking care of her." I smile, inside and out. But now he cautions us—himself, too, it seems. "You don't want to be too optimistic," he says, as though too much hope might break some magic healing spell.

I keep telling Mom how well she's doing, and she keeps smiling in return. It surprises me the way she looks at me. Like *anybody* would. Seeing me, really greeting me with those eyes.

During a break in the doctoring, Mom and I pump out a pretty good rendition of "Pennies From Heaven." Mom smiles, then rubs her hand gently on my face. "You're so happy," she says.

"Yeah, I am. You're doing well, and it's a beautiful day."

July 26 I learned last night that Mom's younger brother Steve is dying of cancer.

July 27 Yesterday I met Emma, a new resident on Mom's hall who is blind but seems to have little, if any, dementia. This evening I stop by her room to visit.

"Hi," I say. "It's Wayne."

"I have no water here," she tells me. I check and she is right, the pitcher is empty and there is no glass or straw.

I get her some water and no sooner do I arrive with it than I hear Nona from the other side of the curtain which separates the two roommates: "I want some water! I want some water!" Her calls are shrill and panicky-sounding, as her verbal communications often are. I cross to her side of the room and find that she has no water, either. "I'll get you some," I assure her even as I hear Emma's voice again, soothed now, reveling, on the other side of the mesh: "Oh, that's so good."

I return with Nona's water, but she is lying on her back in the bed, which is completely flat. "Nona, I'm going to raise the bed so you can sit up some," I explain as I flop the handle into position and begin turning the crank. But I am inexperienced, it seems, and Nona, like a flight instructor guiding home the passenger-pilot in an emergency landing, steps in to fine-tune my effort.

"More . . ." she encourages, ". . . more . . . more . . . that's enough!"

Safely on the tarmac now, I offer the glass of cool liquid and Nona drinks eagerly.

Emma calls out, "You're the nicest person that's come in this room all day!"—quenched thirst makes for an avid admirer—"Could I have some Kleenex? It's here somewhere." I scrabble around in the dim light, find the box, and pass it to her. "Thank you," she says as I hustle back to Nona and start cranking her bed back down to its original position. But again I presume.

"No, no, no!" she yells, as though the bed might explode if I take it an inch lower. "Leave it up a little bit."

I reverse motion, crank slowly, heeding her instructions: "Little more . . . little more . . . that's good." Again her guidance is on target. The bed ends up precisely midway between flat and the drinking angle she originally requested.

Back to Emma now, who is searching by feel for the call button. I find it and give it to her, confident that she is one of the few residents who understands what it is for and how to use it, then fulfill one last request before I leave: to adjust her sheets and blanket which have pulled and rumpled uncomfortably.

Two people, desperate for water and a few minor comforts. I find it an immensely discouraging fact, and an immensely satisfying opportunity as well. A quenching of my own thirst.

July 30 My aunt says that I should decide whether or not to tell my mother about her brother Steve's impending death. Whatever I think is best. It is a quick and easy decision—I will not tell her— but one which brings me no comfort.

Mom's always been close to her brother and, like any human being, she has a right to such information about someone near and dear to her. But I also know I could tell her, sadden her, and a month from now, or a day or an hour, she might remember nothing, or just a nagging remnant. She can't "go through" a grief process. If I tell her once, I'll have to tell her over and over. She will have to grieve, over and over.

August 1, Year Four This evening I do not see a single aide in the facility who is a Meadowlark employee. All I see are "temporaries" from the employment agency. However noble the intentions or vigorous the efforts of these temporary replacement personnel, they are subject to dangerous error at every turn. They do not know the rhythms of the place, the personalities and idiosyncratic behaviors of their charges. Many do not know each other's names, much less the names and needs of those they are here to serve. My mother-in-law is one of four Helens here. I don't think any of them would recognize their last names.

August 6   At the Care Conference, Mom's weight is reported as 102 lbs, surely the least she's ever weighed since childhood.

I keep quiet for a change, and Terry represents her Mom in an effective, balanced way: forceful without being pushy; not complaining, but not passive, either.

"I want my mother to have water at every meal," she says.

"This is a difficult change for people to make," Mindy says. "We're working on it."

And still I keep my mouth shut. Barely.

August 8   Terry is ill today. I arrive at Meadowlark just fifteen minutes before Mom's CWT appointment to find her still in bed, and in a heavier sleep than I've ever seen her. In fact, I'm uncertain whether she is alive, and have to stare at her for many seconds, holding my own breath to mute its sound and still my own body's movement, to know that she is breathing. She is difficult to rouse, although often just the passage of my shadow over her face wakens her.

But within three minutes after she does open her eyes, the aides appear and have her up, dressed, and in her chair. She looks spry, is verbal in small ways on the way over to the clinic, and in the waiting room plucks a magazine from my hands and pages through it herself.

The wound is still closing on the surface and not much improved below, but the tissues remain clean and healthy looking. Dr. Barnes is very friendly, as usual, and shakes my hand. It feels like a supportive family here and the appointments have evolved into a recurring bright spot on our calendar. Something which I would not have predicted five months ago.

During our regular stop at the cafeteria, Mom is wholly at ease. I can leave her parked anywhere and she sits as though she lives there, studying the world.

August 11 This evening I find her asleep, one teddy bear tight in the crook of her arm. She is breathing the way I do when I'm sick or very exhausted, with a greater exhale than inhale, or so it seems. If it keeps up, will this slow-motion panting not run her out of air, out of life, altogether?

August 12 "You don't know what I'm thinking about," my mother says, lying in bed and looking very at ease. Such a long sentence to tempt and tease me with!

"No, I don't. Do you want to tell me?"

"Yes."

Wayne comes in and tapes a few pictures to the wall where Mom can see them when she lies on her right side. In a nursing home, it seems, every detail is a strategy.

"Do you want to tell me about it?" I ask again. She gazes out the window. "Do you want Wayne to leave?"

"Yes."

Wayne obliges.

"Does it have something to do with Dad?"

"Yes," she says, managing somehow to sweeten her smile.

"Did you see Dad today?" The question comes out of an unknown place within, surprising me if not Mom.

"Yes."

She looks out the window again.

"Was it kind of like a dream? A fantasy thing?"

"Yes."

"Did Dad talk to you?"

"Yes."

"What did he say?"

Again her gaze slips beyond the glass. I'm certain that she does this sometimes when she doesn't know what to say, or when she's already forgotten what we're talking about. Is that what's going on here? I'm not sure.

I decide to let her in on a re-framing of our relationship that I've been working on. "You know, we've become really good friends," I say.

Her brow furrows and her face hardens a little. I retreat. I'm not her caregiver; I'm not her friend. I'm her daughter; she's my mother.

"You just want me to be your daughter, don't you,"—she warms me with her smile—"and you're my mom."

I'm going to stop demanding of myself that I know all the answers. She's the one in charge. I may think I'm in charge, but I'm not. This is her life, her body, her disease. Even when decisions have to be made, it may be that she's been making them far more than Wayne and I have. I realize as I sit here with her this day that, looking at it from a bigger, broader perspective, I have to ask myself, "What do I know about it?"

Daughter to mother to caregiver to friend to daughter. I've come full circle.

Mom has been quiet as I think these thoughts. She seems pleased with herself and her situation, and perhaps her daughter, too.

"Your father would want to be here," she says suddenly.

I remember that she spoke the same words in the attorney's office three years ago. She was right then. And she is right now. He would want to be here. And she has wanted him to be with her, too, has longed for him, has waited for him. . . .

I slip an old audiotape "letter" into the player, one that Mom sent to Wayne and me years ago. A decade slips away like magic and her vibrant contralto fills the room, telling us about how my dad gave her an engagement ring in 1938, and how sorry she was that she couldn't wear it to work right away because it needed to have some diamonds set. We listen to the tape together now, Mom and I, touching and admiring her sixty year old wedding ring, turning it to catch the sun.

"Your engagement ring is lost," I say softly, sharing with my mother the secret I have carried for nine months.

"I know," she says.

Two words.

Enough.

29

Love it the way it is.

—Thaddeus Golas

August 13, Year Four My mother-in-law has finished eating and a new aide is offering her juice. "Fluids are the most important thing," she tells her.

There is no water at Mom's table. And so I tell the aide, in a friendly, it's-never-occurred-to-me-to-mention-this-before tone, that Mom likes water, that sometimes a straw is helpful, sometimes it is not. "Oh, I'm glad you told me that," she says.

In the context of our nine-months-and-counting water campaign, her comment strikes me as mildly funny, as though a dark-humored prankster has put these words in her mouth to tease me. But that's not it at all. She's just new. New, and young, and inexperienced, and brimming with sincerity and good will. And I love her for it.

August 28 My mother's eighty-first birthday. Cards and gifts, flowers, friends, family and food. She enjoys every minute. It's as satisfying to Wayne and me as any birthday we've shared with her.

September 12 Dr. Barnes opens her wound a little, finishes his work quickly. When he says goodbye to all of us he tells Wayne and me to take care of her. "And you take care of them," he charges Mom with a smile and the playful wag of his finger. Her eyes sparkle.

There are many kinds of healing intervention.

October 7 While we are playing Mom's *South Pacific* CD, Margaret, the retired nurse who lives down the hall, appears at the doorway, her body hunched over her walker, her face strained with real or imagined worries.

"Come join us," Wayne says, waving her in.

A hint of smile. "It's so nice to have people who share a feeling for music," she says.

Soon she is swaying to the strains of "Some Enchanted Evening." We sing together, the four of us. Margaret is happy, talking, singing. An old friend.

October 9 The milk thing just goes on and on. Terry's mother has received milk four or five times that we're aware of in the past week, and still doesn't receive water consistently. Mindy says that she will follow the corporate policy of providing milk unless there is a doctor's order to the contrary. So a week ago Terry had the doctor write an order: "No milk products during allergy season." It got written on her diet card, but nobody knew what it meant—who's going to decide when it's allergy season? Terry called the doctor again. She said she would call Meadowlark and clarify that her order is for year-round implementation.

But tonight Mom is served milk. When I mention to the aide, Mary Beth, that Mom isn't supposed to have milk she wonders aloud, "Why do they keep bringing it out?"

My question, too. Milk in hand, I go in search of kitchen staff to find an answer to this ancient riddle. The young woman at the serving window explains that Mom gets milk because her diet card specifies milk. The kitchen has received two orders to discontinue milk, she tells me, but apparently this is not enough. "I have to do what the card says," she tells me.

She refers me to Lily, who actually filled the milk order today. I know Lily. Very down-to-earth. Very approachable.

I enter the kitchen inner sanctum, find Lily washing dishes, and broach the subject amidst billows of Clorox-laced steam. I hold out

Mom's glass, explaining tongue-in-cheek that I have brought it as a visual aid.

"You can just dump it there in the sink," she says. I do as she instructs, but tell her I am hoping for a somewhat longer-term solution. She gives me the same story: it has to be changed on the card; only Mindy can change the card. "But," she adds, just as the final embers of my hope are fading, "I can do it if I get a pink slip from Nursing."

"The doctor has already called twice," I assure her as she opens the wash unit, removes a tray of clean dishes, and slides a batch of dirty in its place.

"Maybe so. But I have to get a pink slip from Nursing."

"A pink slip. . . . You know, the gal out at the serving window said she's got two orders of some kind."

"No, I have to have a pink slip."

I leave the kitchen and find the evening nurse. "I thought that was all taken care of," she says in response to my sad tale.

"A lot of people kind of know about it, I guess, but I'm told they need a pink slip."

She searches diligently through a stack of paper, through mounds of looseleaf folders, through drawers, but apparently does not find whatever it is she's looking for. But she does find phone-in orders from the doctor. She shows me one: No Milk Products.

"Okay. Here's what they need." She produces the prized pink slip, writes No Milk Products, and signs it. She walks the twenty paces to the kitchen window, knocks, and hands it to someone inside. When she returns she says to me, "She told me they have three of these now."

"Who told you that?" I ask, feeling that my good name and credibility have been dragged through spilled milk.

"I don't know. I don't know the people back there," she says, but from her description I surmise that it was June, whom I also know and like quite well.

I trot back to the kitchen, find June, and replay the story for her. She listens patiently then says to me, not unpleasantly but in a way so as to indicate she believes English might be my third language, "We have three of these now."

"You do? Three?" I hold up three fingers. June looks at them.

"What I'm saying to you is, Nursing has done its part."

On my way out I meet up with the first young lady, the one who told me of the "two orders" originally. She shows them to me: one for allergy season dated Oct. 1, one from last night for No Milk Products, and the one that was delivered minutes ago. Pink slips all.

June joins us now and boldly places a piece of tape over the "milk" section on Mom's diet card. "No Milk Products," she writes on the tape. We brainstorm non-milk desserts, side dishes, and snacks: applesauce, canned fruits, bananas, toast. June says that she has noticed that Mom receives orange juice quite frequently—she receives it at virtually every meal, in fact—and to the exclusion of available alternatives. "Doesn't she like other kinds?" she asks.

"She loves apple juice," I tell her. "And cranberry, too."

"I wouldn't want to have orange juice at every meal," June says. "We'll rotate them."

We're on a roll.

— 30 —

Nearly all of my patients, so it seems to me, whatever their problems, reach out to life—and not only despite their conditions, but often because of them, and even with their aid.

—Oliver Sacks, M.D.

"It's a lovely night."

—Helen

October 13, Year Four   Mom is whimpering, even as she watches *Going My Way* and laughs. During a break from the video she says, "I want to say something to you," then makes garbled sounds that neither Wayne nor I can make anything of.

"What did you say?" I ask.

She repeats the whole thing in the tiniest, most ancient, crackling voice I've ever heard. "I want to say something to you. . . . It's . . . a lovely night."

October 14   Renee calls. Mom had a temperature during the night of 101.8, although now at mid-morning it is 99.6. The doctor has ordered blood work and a shot of antibiotics.

Wayne and I are getting ready to go on a school tour at the end of the month. And although we've arranged for our friend April to visit Mom while we're away, her elevated temperature raises unsettling questions: Is this serious? Is she dying?

We don't want her to die before or during this trip. It would be inconvenient. It's hard to feel okay about such a thought, even though it's perfectly understandable: things affect us. We've been working hard to keep our business alive. This trip is an important part of that effort. Mom's temperature last night was the highest that we're aware of since her arrival at Meadowlark. Suddenly we're thinking about mortuaries and cremation, and what we'd do with ashes, and announcements in the paper. The mind works in unsettling ways.

October 20 "Your mom understands a lot," Margaret says to me. "You can see it in her eyes. She knows what's going on."

"You are right, Margaret."

"I'm an old RN," she reminds me.

October 24 At CWT Dr. Barnes notes that the wound has completely closed. He guesses that some tunneling still remains beneath the surface but we all discuss the matter together and agree on his suggestion not to open it back up, to follow her body's lead and give it a try this way instead. We'll bring her back in one month.

October 25 A huge snowstorm has delayed our trip for several days, with level depths of 16-30 inches across the eastern half of the state. Denver International and essentially every road in eastern Colorado are closed. Fifteen-foot drifts are reported on I-70.

Worried that Meadowlark may be operating with far too few staff, I arrive in our old four-wheel-drive International to assure myself that Mom is okay and to help out otherwise if needed.

"Where's that wife of yours?" Lucille calls to me before I've stomped the snow from my shoes on the mat inside the door. "She's at home, writing a book," I tell her. She rolls closer and hands me a long-stemmed rose. "Give this to her when you see her," she says.

On a larger scale, too, things are going well. The mood in the place is good, and Mom seems fine. She eats some and I feed her some; she drinks some and she dribbles some; her nose runs some, she sits crooked some, and she smiles some.

November 5 Today Wayne and I have returned from our school visits in the Midwest. In the space of a week we've made nearly two dozen presentations, sold hundreds of books, and roamed through the lands of imagination and adventure with more than 2,500 children. After this short absence, Mom and the other residents here seem older, more ill, than before.

The young and the old—I am fortunate to spend so much time with both groups. So different, yet so similar in the ease with which I connect with them. Despite the occasional public clamor over this or that issue affecting them, both groups are essentially off society's radar, yet both are eager for respectful attention, both so able and willing to connect at an authentic level, both as refreshing and rejuvenating as wind off high mountain snow.

November 12 So emaciated is Terry's mother that, lying here in the bed, the skin above her clavicle sags into a deep, dark hollow that runs from neck to shoulder. I cannot see the bottom, and wonder for one unsettling moment if there is none; if I am looking at another wound, an actual hole to the inside of her. The bizarre illusion quickly passes, but not before driving home an undeniable fact: physically, little remains of my mother-in-law.

A new aide, Marilyn, helps Mom out of bed. She ends up all crooked and contorted in the chair. Marilyn notices this, and together she and I work on straightening her, but we are unsuccessful. It is hard for me to accept this failure in so elementary a task, to see Mom slumped forward, one leg sticking out to the side as though to trip an unwary passer-by.

After a while we try again, this time with limited success. Her right leg is so contracted that her foot is up almost onto the seat. She's tiny and frail, yet her legs are like vises and cannot be undone.

I thank Marilyn for her extra efforts. "It wasn't that much," she says. "That's what we're here for."

November 14 After she finishes eating, Terry and I take Mom to the hall. "Do you want to wait out here," I ask her as she sips her orange juice, "or go in there, to your room?" A two-choice question. My mistake.

"Yes," she says.

"Out here?" I ask, voicing my preference.

"No. In my room."

She has indicated ownership of the room where she lives. She has vetoed my suggested choice. She has not only remembered but understood and selected from the options of my compound question two exchanges back.

No. In my room. Four remarkable words.

November 15   Leah, who sits across from my mother at the feeding table, is hardly ever awake, or so it seems. I have never heard her talk. She eats only what is placed into her mouth by others. Most of the time she doesn't seem to be in our world any longer.

Today she sits there, tiny and bundled as a puppy in a Christmas stocking. Her eyes are open. She is smiling at me.

As is her usual posture, she is slid far down in her chair, much further than Mom has ever been. She sits now at the table almost on her back. Her body is always tight and contracted. Today is no different. Her left hand is clenched in a fist. Her thumb, clamped between her fore and middle fingers, protrudes slightly, like the stolen nose in the trick for small children.

As I sit here with my mom, talking to her, feeding her, I occasionally catch Leah's eye and smile at her. In many conversations I have here at Meadowlark, words are of secondary importance; in some, like now, they are absent altogether.

I send a little wave to Leah, a private, rippling-finger wave, skimming to her just above the tabletop. Moments later her forefinger releases its grip on her thumb ever so slightly, then cuts a silent, tiny arc of perhaps a single inch through the air.

It is a small, secret movement. Yet it is a wave, as surely as my own.

November 16 I lean over the bed as my mother touches my hair and face, just keeps rubbing her hands on me, stroking my mouth and my cheeks, my teeth, now back into my hair; all the while smiling with incredible joy, as though she were meeting her daughter after a very long separation.

November 17 My mother-in-law, parked at the table forty minutes before the scheduled start of dinner, has her bib stretched out in front of her, and is working to get it nice and straight and free of wrinkles.

I come in quietly, slowly entering her range of vision from the side. She senses me, turns her head, sees me fully. A grin spreads from ear to ear. She stutters like an old engine on a cold morning.

"Feeer . . . Fer gosh sakes!"

An aide approaches, smiles at Mom and says something to her in sweet tones.

"Oh, gudsluenls, dhe sdlgud guys saaksid lbirncrds an osgslsk!" Mom tells her.

Neither I nor the aide can get much of it, except maybe the word "guys." She smiles at Mom. They both seem content with that.

November 18 After supper I take my mother-in-law out to the lobby. We are barely settled when Vic approaches in his wheelchair.

Before I ever met him, before I ever talked to him, I was warned about Vic. "Watch out," I was told, "he's a dangerous one." I took the caution to heart. Lean and grizzled, he seemed possessed of a wiry strength and steely will that might combine to wallop someone pretty good if he took a mind to do so. Our first interaction consisted of me extending my hand, and his taking it in his iron grip, after he had fallen out of his wheelchair. "Thanks," he said.

In the months since that day, each time I see him I greet him, offer my hand again, and we renew and strengthen some mysterious bond that links us. Our conversations are typically short and vague, and carry little literal meaning. But they form a bridge between us, a road that carries the commerce of caring and connectedness, the simple enjoyment of each other's company.

I have no expectations of Vic, nor does he of me. I neither fear his judgment, nor seek his approval. I know of no interests or activities we might have shared had we met in Vic's more vigorous past. We do not argue or debate, or make any effort to impress one another. We do not lament the state of the larger world, neither do we burden one another with the state of our personal psychic or physical worlds. I do not know Vic's last name; he has never learned my first. In a lifetime of nearly fifty years, I have met a great many people. A few of those have become friends. Vic is one.

This evening he is obviously a man on a mission. He rolls toward Mom, head on, but stops as he comes abreast of me.

"Could I talk to this lady?" he asks me.

Conversations with Vic don't usually make this much literal sense. "It's okay with me if it's okay with her," I tell him, not entirely certain of the proper etiquette for chaperoning one's eighty-one year old mother-in-law. Mom ignores us both.

Vic rolls forward slowly, until the footrests of their chairs touch. He looks directly into her face. "Now I'm not going to say very many words," he tells her, "but you're a very beautiful lady. Your skin is very smooth."

Mom averts her eyes.

"I see she's losing a little interest," Vic says to me. His quest has my respect and my moral support but I think it best to give nothing more than a sympathetic tilt of my head.

Speaking again to Mom, he says, "I guess I said too many words." He waits a brief moment for a response that does not come, then backs his chair two feet. Again he looks at me.

"Maybe that was enough for now," I tell him quietly.

Without another word, my friend pivots and rolls away.

November 20 Mom's wound is still closed and looking healthy. Dr. Barnes is pleased, and a little incredulous. "How'd we do that?" he wonders aloud.

One more appointment, in a month. Just to make sure.

November 21   While cleaning the porch I come across my mother's boots. Brown, mid-calf, dusty now and incorporated into the webbing of some industrious spider. They don't fit me. They aren't worth giving away. I know that Mom won't be wearing them again, but I cannot throw them out because . . .

Even though she weighs 95 pounds, and has been sitting in a wheelchair for a year, and long ago forgot how to walk, and her legs are badly contracted . . .

Because what kind of daughter throws out her mother's only boots?

What if she needs them?

31

"I've got a cannibal on my back."

—Vic

November 25, Year Four The social worker calls to say that they would like to—need to, she corrects herself—move Terry's mother to another room. "She's in a Medicare room," she explains, and they need Medicare beds for people coming out of the hospital. She tells me it's in Mom's best interest to move because being in a Medicare room now might cause her to lose her eligibility for benefits after any future hospital stay; perhaps a needed hospitalization itself might not be covered. They don't need a bed right now, she tells me, or in the imminent future. They're reorganizing their Medicare services. "This is probably all just mumbo-jumbo to you," she says.

I tell her that it is not mumbo-jumbo, but that it is a surprise to hear that Mom is in a Medicare room, insofar as she was moved a year ago to this room, specifically because she couldn't be in a Medicare room.

"Her current room probably wasn't a Medicare room at that time," she says, which only raises in my mind the question of when it became one. The next day? Months ago? Yesterday? Is it in fact a Medicare room now, or is that only a plan?

"What if Mom would have to go to the hospital today?" I ask.

"Well, maybe I'd better stop and back up here, because I guess I don't really know, for certain. I could check about that."

But this does not deter her from proceeding to moving plans. She wants to move Mom to Nona's room.

"When is it you want to do this?" I ask.

"In the next couple of days."

She wants to know how we can proceed, suggests that she could show us the room. Like a real estate agent. Like we have never seen Nona's room before.

I tell her that I need first to share this information with Terry. And that we don't want any move to happen until we have had time to consider the situation, to talk with them about any concerns we might have, and until we have agreed to it. I tell her that a major consideration, as I see it now, is the fact that Mom has lived in this room for a year and that she identifies it—by location, decor, layout, window view—as hers. "And that," I tell her, "is important to us."

"We aren't going to do anything until you're on board with it," she says.

Only marginally reassuring words, insofar as I had a distinctly different impression at the start of the conversation.

November 26   For the past twenty-four hours Terry and I have spent almost full-time researching this room-change situation. We talked to the ombudsman this morning and picked up information on Residents' Rights; we talked to Delta's son, who said that he hasn't been informed of a proposed room change for his mother; we called an attorney, the Medicare contractor in Dallas, and others knowledgeable about the morass of Medicare rules and regulations.

I go in at five, awash in feelings of betrayal and anger after dealing with this all day, and find Mom peaceful and untroubled, placing a delicate kiss on the nose of her teddy bear. I pick her little stuffed mouse off the TV and hand it to her. She lays the bear on the mouse, bumping and rubbing them together.

"Hey, Mom," I say, "what are they doing?"

She looks at me as though I might not be very bright. "They're enjoying themselves," she says.

When I'm with her it's like I've stumbled into an oasis. Maybe a different universe.

Thanksgiving Terry, Mom, and I join other families at one of
the long tables set up in the lobby, just outside the very full dining
room. A festive atmosphere fills the building and food is plentiful.
While we wait to be served, Terry and I both notice Vic in his
wheelchair toward the far end of Mom's hall. Terry encourages me
to see if he wants to join us, even as Drew, an aide, assures us, "No,
he refused. He refused."

"Hey, Vic!" I call, waving to my friend when I am halfway down
the long, empty corridor.

Vic doesn't answer. His body is slack and looped forward. He
stares at the floor.

"Victor, Terry and her mom and I would like to know if you
would honor us by coming and having Thanksgiving dinner with us,"
I say in the playfully formal tone that I often take with Vic.

"I'm ready to go," he says without lifting his head.

But when I get right up next to him I see that he is not ready to
go. "Vic, your brakes are locked up here. I'm going to take the
brakes off." I release the left, then the right, moving deliberately,
cautiously. "Everything okay, Vic?" Something feels wrong.

I start pushing. But Vic is so limp that the rubber soles of his
shoes drag and catch on the tile floor. "Vic, lift your feet," I instruct
and he does, but in a few seconds they drop and catch again. I have
to repeat my request time and again, and push slowly in between so
as not to injure his foot or ankle when he lets them sag.

I have never seen Vic in this condition. I wonder whether he has
had a stroke, although except for his lack of muscle tone and diminished energy he seems himself. It's as though his body's power
switch has been turned to low. Nor does a stroke explain the curious
circumstances in which I found him: alone, parked with brakes
locked, at the far end of a hall in which I have never seen him before, at mealtime—he's always hungry!—on Thanksgiving. It takes
me most of our slow traverse of the corridor to process all this.

As we near the mouth of the hall, Drew approaches again, focused and eager, offering to take Vic off my hands and into the
dining room. I have known Drew for some months and find him to

be a capable, hardworking, and responsible aide. But today I am wary.

"That's all right," I tell Drew, tightening my grip on the handles of Vic's chair. "We invited him to eat with us. We're doing okay." I position Vic at the table next to me, and Terry asks the first aide within earshot if we can get a meal for him. Vic is still slumped forward, his spine curved, his head suspended like heavy fruit on a straining branch, barely above the tabletop.

Drew comes by again barely a minute after our arrival. "You know," he says, "I think it'd be better if we just take him on into the dining room."

"No," I tell him, "that's okay. It would be helpful, though, if we could get his meal as quickly as possible."

"Well, you know, we're really . . . things are kind of falling apart in the kitchen and we're . . . I don't know how fast we can get it to him."

I wonder, not aloud, what might be the urgent purpose then of taking him into the dining room? The question is made moot when the previous aide appears with Vic's meal. We get the food in front of him and, though his chin is in his plate the whole time, Vic is his usual respectful and polite self.

"How're things going?" I ask him. "Can I help you a little bit with this?"

"No-oo," he says, gamely aiming a lone string bean in the general direction of his mouth, ". . . I'm doin' all right. . . . I hope I'm not holdin' you folks up."

"Nope. We're doin' fine. We're all doin' okay." Perhaps a minute passes before I ask again, "How's it goin', Vic?"

"It's goin' slow," he says. ". . . I've got a cannibal on my back."

It goes on like this for half an hour, me fretting all the while and Vic just as polite and sweet as anyone I've ever met. Eventually we finish our meals, Terry and Mom and Vic and I.

Mom is looking fatigued and sleepy; Vic seems to be perking up.

November 29 "Oh, Helen, I'm going to be able to work with you tomorrow," the aide says at the end of her shift.

"That's good," my mother says.

Later, another aide is helping her to bed. She tells me that Mom is awake quite a bit at night.

"Is that something new?" I ask.

"It's been going on for the three or four months that I've been working nights," she says. "I come in and spend time with her."

"Thank you very much," I say.

For four days I've felt like taking my mom out of here, because of this room change business. But I can't move her. She'd be losing too much love. We'll deal with this. If there are battles to be fought, we'll fight them here. At home.

December 3 It's more than an hour past breakfast. My mother-in-law is still at the table but has eaten essentially nothing.

Maybe that's the way she wants to go out, and we shouldn't be trying to . . . I mean, she'll eat when we feed her, but I don't know if she always wants to. Is that a reason to feed somebody who seems happy not eating? To make me happy?

It's a real dilemma. When I see this skinny little person with food in front of her that she doesn't seem to know what to do with, I kind of want to get it in her mouth. Terry and I are constantly walking that line, weighing things in the balance, trying to make decisions for her that human beings usually make for themselves. When they're tired they lie down; when they're hungry they eat.

This is what dying is, short of sudden death, a stroke, an accident. Things stop working. We keep trying to fix them as best we can. We keep losing ground.

I think we ought not to be too hard on ourselves, or on anyone else, for not making everything perfect. We can't circumvent death by feeding her until she gets past the crisis. This is not a crisis. This is every day. Drinking. Swallowing. Breathing.

Terry says she hopes Mom stays happy through all this, because that's the main thing. We've got to keep hold of that.

32

One world at a time.

—Henry David Thoreau

December 6, Year Four My mother is having a bad time in the wheelchair, slipping lower and lower, settling in lumpy fashion, like a sack of potatoes. Jody, the former volunteer who's hired on as an aide now, helps me straighten her, but Mom's legs are an unfixable problem and ten minutes later she is sagged way down again. She is tired, and practically out of the chair altogether.

"Do you want me to get someone to help you get into bed?" I ask her.

"Yes."

I find Jody and when she and her helper come Mom tells them and anyone who has ears to hear, "It's a fine day."

In the hall, I put on my coat while they put her to bed, feeling guilty about leaving before I see her all tucked in. Jody finds me hesitating in the hallway. "Oh, we'll tuck her in," she assures with a smile that warms me.

But on the drive home, in the cold car, I worry. Did they give her her little bears to hold?

December 18 At CWT, Dr. Barnes is all smiles. The new skin has matured and looks even healthier than a month ago. "A healing like this is very unusual," he tells us.

He discharges her. It's been forty-one weeks.

December 22 In the days following the social worker's phone call about the room change, Terry and I amassed a considerable amount of information concerning Medicare benefits and nursing home residents' rights regarding room assignments. We learned that Medicare coverage of hospital services will not be affected by Mom's continued residence in a Medicare-certified room. We learned also that, while her post-hospitalization benefits might or might not be affected—there are arguable points on both sides of the issue—it doesn't matter to us in any practical sense. We don't see physical or occupational therapies as a likely part of her future, nor the need for any nursing care more specialized or intensive than she now receives. And we learned that, whatever Medicare benefits she might lose, the choice of whether to put them at risk remains hers. She cannot be forced to accept a room change.

Bolstered by this knowledge, we decided weeks ago that we are not going to budge on this. As far as we're concerned, Mom's room is her home for the rest of her life. We have waited to see what might be Meadowlark's next step, but have heard not one further word on the subject. We think the move issue is over. If it is not, we're prepared.

December 24 Renee calls. They suspected a urinary tract infection, sent out a sample, which has come back positive. Mom's doctor has started her on an antibiotic. I thank Renee and wish her a happy Christmas. And then begin to worry about my mother.

December 25 For some reason there was no Family Christmas Dinner planned this year, so Terry and I requested a space where we and her mother could share a special lunch together. We've ended up in a small, windowless storage room, squeezed in among a few sticks of unwanted furniture and a small mountain of gaily wrapped packages. Our tabletop is stained and dusty and there is barely room for the three of us to wedge in around it.

Cramped though we are and sleepy though Mom is, we're doing our best to make our meal a Christmas celebration, and I decide that now is the time for the simple toast I have planned. I quickly fill Terry's glass and mine with sparkling apple cider, saving Mom's—in deference to her weakened condition a tiny, plastic, one-ounce medication cup—for last. Terry places the little container of golden bubbles in her mother's hand. I raise my glass in salute. "To Helen—"

The sound of her name focuses Mom's attention on me, our eyes meet, and I feel the beginnings of a small, proud smile forming the corners of my mouth. Our three glasses still poised in air, I raise my cup an inch higher and extend it toward Mom.

"To you, Mom," I start again.

Before I can say another word, she reaches out with her free hand and plucks the proffered glass from my grasp. Both hands laden with drinks now, Mom brings this newest one to her lips and gracefully drains it.

December 27   Lucille wheels away from her table and rolls over to my mother's. She finds a spot right across from her and parks herself there. The aides keep trying to coax her back to her own table and she just keeps shaking her head. Finally, they bring her food over and she eats her breakfast with us at the feeding table.

In the hallway outside my mother's room I come upon Irma, a newer resident whom I have already come to love, sitting in her chair in the hall, facing the wall. "Mama," she calls softly. When I come near she grabs my hand. I get on one knee and she hugs me to her, right to her chest. She lets me go and then I lean in again and she holds me again. With both her arms, holds on tight.

I love what happens in this place. I hug Irma because it is in my human nature to do so. And Irma hugs me for this same reason. I am being hugged as much as I am hugging.

Before my mother's illness, I might have thought that dementia constituted the supreme barrier to relationship. But my experience with her, and with Irma, and with so many people here, has demonstrated just the opposite. I know that Irma will accept my hug, without interpretation or judgment. I know that with her I am good enough just as I am in this moment, and that confidence allows me to reach out to her, to experience the human connection that is simply, already, there. The real barrier to relationship, it seems, is thought. The judgment, doubt, fear, and score-keeping that our busy brains so easily fall into. Dementia lessens those interferences, or eliminates them altogether. Dementia, it seems to me, facilitates the recognition and experience of true relationship.

January 2 Mom is tired and phlegmy and sneezing. The fellow who usually sits next to her at the table is in bed. When I last saw him, a few days ago, he was looking terribly ill. Another resident has died. The dining room looks half empty.

Wayne and another family member meet with the director of nurses and her assistant for about an hour and a half today. They do a good job, I think, exploring ways to build community across all groups here—all the levels of workers, the families, the residents. I think that's a beautiful thing to keep putting out in front of people.

January 4 My mother-in-law's roommate Delta is in bed. A tube delivering oxygen snakes across the blankets, down to where it connects to the machine on the floor. She looks very ill.

"She's sick," the aide tells me.

"What's wrong?"

"It's cancer." I detect an uneasiness in her voice. Perhaps she has gone beyond the professional limit of sharing, perhaps the cancer frightens her. "Oh, she'll get better," she assures. "We're nursing her."

Yes, they surely are. But does the cancer know?

January 7 I push my mother-in-law's chair out to the sunroom and we watch the snow, fluttering past our eyes like cottonwood seeds. Bill, our "resident poet," puts out his hand and catches her attention. "I just want to shake your hand," he says. "You're a beautiful lady."

Mom weighs ninety pounds. Her sparse, white hair is cut very short. She looks frail and sick. It must be the beatific smile she wears most of the time now that he and others are so drawn to. We go back to her room, the aides put her to bed, and minutes later she is in a heavy sleep.

I learn as I am leaving the nursing home that Delta has just died. Terry and I have seen more people die in the past twelve months than in both our lifetimes prior to that. I don't know how these young workers handle it, month after month.

The social worker asks if I want Mom to be removed from the room during the post-mortem preparation. "No," I tell her. "She's asleep, and she's so tired. Besides, she takes things pretty well in stride."

I don't know exactly what is going to transpire, though. I don't want to leave Mom alone. I decide to sit with her for a bit and find that, sound asleep though she's been, she is suddenly awake. Striving for a gentle, matter-of-fact tone, I tell her that Delta—I consciously choose not to refer to her as "your roommate"—has died, that she was very old and had gotten sick with cancer.

Mom sleeps most of the time during the next hour. The aides come in to clean and prepare Delta's body, arrange it in the freshened bed. There are at least three, sometimes four aides in the room. They work efficiently under the harsh light of the fluorescent tubes beyond the curtain; busy, in hushed tones, yet unavoidably noisy in a new and tiny universe where any sound at all seems too much. Twice they bump Mom's bed, move it an inch across the floor; Delta's trash can rattles a small death knell. With each disturbance Mom flutters awake. I greet her with a smile and a soft hello and she soon slips back to sleep.

When the aides are finished they disappear like dew, and in an instant the room grows entirely quiet. I slip to Delta's side. Her body suddenly looks like simply that, a thing more gaunt, more pallid than ever Delta was; the eyes a thin line of pearl gray between almost-closed lids, the jaw slack. I wish that I had recognized that she was so near death when I saw her only minutes before her passing, wish that I had spent some special moment with her.

The undertaker appears at the door, trailing a narrow, shiny stretcher. I sit with Mom, look up as he lingers there, just noticing him really, in a moment of stilled time. Suddenly I read in his eye his silent question: Is this the body I seek? With a word and a gesture, I direct him to Delta's side of the room. I pull Mom's privacy curtain all the way, so that she is surrounded, protected. Within three or four minutes he has placed Delta's body in a corduroy body bag. Will she emerge from her cocoon, I wonder, into some new and unimagined life?

Mom wakes just as the gurney rolls out the door. She gives me a questioning look and I fear for a moment that perhaps I have made the wrong decision about leaving her in the room. I lean over her and point to the closed curtain. "I did that," I say with no further explanation. She smiles at my accomplishment, then falls back asleep.

I quietly slide the fabric open, and think back on the past hour. I am very positively impressed with the aides: those who prepared the body, the several who came in to spend a few moments with it beforehand, and others after. The depth of their emotion has been considerable, and obvious to me. One or two I think didn't come in, only because their emotions were too strong to allow it. I feel a companionship with all the aides, a renewed and deepened respect for the difficulty of the job they do with so little recognition and for so little financial compensation.

Although only minutes have passed since the undertaker's departure, I see Mary Beth—the first at Delta's bedside after her death, and who spent the longest time there—moving down the hall, scooping up ice for the water pitchers in the rooms, serving the needs of others.

I gaze at Mom—a mere swell of blanket, white fleece upon the pillow, guardian bear tight against her chest—then raise my eyes a fraction to the empty, still bed beneath the window. This end will come for her too. It could be weeks, or months, or years away; it could come tomorrow. I've known this before now, of course, but the events of this lovely, somber, snowy morning, have made it so much more real.

33

"We can get anything we want in here."

—Helen

January 9, Year Four   So many people dying. Delta just two days ago, and today Hazel, who made it through not quite six months of her second century.

January 11   My mother is Buddha at the dining table. Perfectly erect, eyes closed. Nothing but a smooth expanse of empty tabletop in front of her.

I touch her arm lightly. She opens her eyes and looks at me, a smile slowly lighting her face, like the glow of the hidden moon as it nears the feathered edge of a cloud.

A new aide tells me what a beautiful person my mother is. "She doesn't talk much," the young lady adds, as though pointing out a minor flaw I might want to attend to.

January 15   Such a precarious balance. Two days ago, my mother-in-law started having trouble drinking. Yesterday evening it was the same. She tried to drink, but could barely lift the plastic glass to her lips. And when she succeeded at that, she couldn't get it aligned to her mouth or tilt it correctly. Her eyes were half closed. She tried to eat, tried to take food from me when I placed it in her mouth, but she couldn't swallow right. Every time I gave her any liquid half of it ran down her chin. She couldn't suck on the straw. I talked to Kamilah, the new evening nurse on Mom's hall, and asked her to do a urinalysis. "We only do that in an emergency," she said. "Or if you insist." It was the first time we had ever spoken to one another. I don't know if I insisted or not.

Today Mom looks much better. She's drinking water efficiently; sitting ramrod straight at the table, with an almost aristocratic bearing; begins feeding herself when her pancakes arrive. Her nose is running and I give her a Kleenex. "Thank you," she says, and then blows her nose, something I haven't seen her do in months.

Terry and I return after lunch—less than four hours have passed—to find Mom in her room, sitting in her chair, shivering uncontrollably. She has a temperature of 100.2.

At supper an aide feeds her, but she looks stronger and more alert than at noon. She's eating and drinking pretty well, even reaching out toward the food. Kamilah tells me her temperature is 100.8 degrees, higher than earlier.

Such a precarious balance.

January 23   Sharon calls to tell me she woke from a nap, certain that she should come to see our mother. She and her daughter Mimi will be here at the end of February.

January 24   I show Mom some photographs, always a pleasant pastime for her. She likes one of her and Wayne so much that she props it up in her scrambled eggs and looks at it while she eats.

January 27   "Sip, Mom. Don't chew, sip." I take the straw from my mother's mouth, mime the proper action, then give it back again. I repeat the process until, after several failed attempts, she suddenly gets the hang of it and drains the glass.

At supper she eats her mashed potatoes with her fingers, then does the same with pureed peas, which is a less productive venture. Her hands are a mess and she doesn't like it. I clean them, but seconds later she is eating again with her fingers.

January 28   After visiting with Mom this evening, Terry and I go out into the hall while Jody puts Mom to bed. In just those few minutes I talk with Kamilah, Marilyn, Mark, Henry, Margaret, Lucille, Nona, and Vic. I return to Mom's room with this simple but distinct feeling: I like it here. Not all the time, but there is a part of me—a part growing for many months now—that feels immense affection, not only for Mom but for many other residents and for the staff, and even for this geographical place I have come to so often and which I know so well.

Mom has a life here, and I am part of it.

February 3 Marilyn is feeding Mom at supper and Mom is resisting her, fending her off with her spoon, which Marilyn seems to be taking with humor. "We're having sword fights," she jokes.

Mom isn't in an eating mode. She's in a move-everything-around-on-the-plate-and-flatten-it-out mode. Despite a year of steady effort by Terry and me, there is no water at her place.

February 6 Margaret, the old RN, has moved into Mom's room. I cannot think of two more suited roommates.

Marilyn tells me that earlier today, when she peeked into the room to wave and say hi to her, Mom smiled and volunteered, "We can get anything we want in here." Marilyn got a big boost out of that, as I do now from her telling.

February 10 I tell Mom about a talk I had with her brother Joe and that he mentioned their childhood dog. "Well, I'll be damned!" she exclaims. I wonder aloud whether Perry Como is still singing anymore. "I doubt it," she says.

February 11 My mother-in-law has been talking since I got here. Twenty minutes of conversation. I can't understand most of what she is saying, but she is clearly making statements, not just mumblings or even single word responses. In fact, most of them have been initiated by her rather than responses to me, and they are long sentences with even the subtle rhythms of conversational speech.

Several staff have been telling me they've experienced the same thing recently, but this is the most extreme example I've seen.

I call Terry and tell her about what's happening and then put Mom on. I am struck by how intently she focuses on the sounds coming into her ear through the tiny and physically unfamiliar hardware of the portable phone. She speaks long phrases of words I can't understand. Now she listens. I hear Terry say, "I love you."

Suddenly Mom's eyes narrow in concentration, her lips quiver and dance. The muscles in her throat tense and relax, then tense again. She wants to speak, and though seconds have elapsed and no sound has emerged, it is obvious to me that not only the thoughts but the words themselves are there, somewhere. It is as though her brain has been sending complex instructions for the physical manufacture of words in her larynx. They are being laboriously transported now to her mouth and lips. I can imagine them, jiggling along toward freedom like the little cylinders of ice in a garden hose turned on in the morning sun after a night of frost.

Finally, the words—words we haven't heard in a year—are born, pushed out into the world, every syllable a tightly focused struggle, a special effort: "I . . . lo . . . ve . . . you."

February 14   As soon as Mom gets up for the Valentine's Day party she is exhausted. She can hardly eat or drink. Running on empty.

Wayne arrives bearing two roses, one for Mom and one for me. She twists and twists the rose stem, until she is able to bend and, finally, break it. And then she tries to eat it.

February 16   My mother-in-law is withdrawn, distant, looking past me. There's been a very big change in her over the past four or five days.

Irma usually eats at Mom's table. Today she isn't here. I visit her briefly in her room and she looks tiny and weak, extraordinarily different than the last time I saw her a few days ago. It has taken that long for me to even register that she's not been at her usual place at the table. It upsets me that I'm so unaware.

I don't think Irma is going to recover.

February 18   Josie's here to take Mom for her shower. But she doesn't just wheel her away, she salutes her. Mom loves it, actually laughs, and this is all the encouragement Josie requires. Seeing the success of a right-handed salute, she raises her left hand and snaps it away sharply. Mom slaps her thigh in appreciation. Josie salutes with both hands now and kicks her legs out in march rhythm. It's very physical, slapstick stuff that doesn't strike me as all that funny, but what does get me going is watching Mom, who is beside herself. She smiles, the smile turns into a grin, and the grin gets bigger and bigger with every passing second. She makes no sound, no "Ha ha ha," but sound or no, whatever it is that we call laughter, that's what she is doing.

She is out of control now, rocking forward and back, miming her laugh like an actor in a silent movie. It's a fun, funny scene, that just keeps building on itself for a long and glorious minute until, finally, Terry and I are laughing, too. Sound and all.

February 19   Irma has died.

February 20   My mother-in-law has received a packet of certified letters from a law office in California. Official-looking envelopes with embossed lettering and 6-line return addresses. There are four of them, nearly identical.

I open the first one here at Mom's table and scan it quickly. Foreclosure details on her mobile home. I'm not surprised. We discontinued payments on the debt-burdened property long ago and gave permission for the park authorities to rent it out and keep the receipts to cover the lot rent. These letters are nothing more than the final closing of a door we passed through two years ago. In different circumstances such papers might be a source of great distress.

But we are past that. These pages bring closure and, though not without a touch of poignancy, relief.

I lay the letter aside, intending to study the lot of them later. But Mom spots the pile and starts a slow, labored reach for it, her arm, hand, and fingers unfolding at each joint to give her a range that somehow surprises me. Finally, she snags one of the thick envelopes and drags it off the stack toward her. For a fleeting moment I am unnerved, as though she might read these pages of legalese and take umbrage at the outrageous revelations they contain.

She studies the envelope, points to the return address—**Law Offices of Rockford & Faire**. "Rockford Files," she says, then slides her finger to the second name. "Fair . . . Lady." I point to her name on the envelope, in much smaller print. "Helen," she says. I move my finger to her last name. She makes a sound or two but no word that I can recognize.

I open the letter, shifting the page toward her so that we both can see it. "These are letters about your mobile home," I say. "Everything is being taken care of." I point to names in the first paragraph, the people who are taking legal title to her once-precious home. "They'll be paying all the bills," I translate. I fold the page in thirds, slide it back into its envelope. "Remember how a while back you asked me to take care of all that stuff?"

"Yes," she says.

"Well, I have. Everything is going fine."

February 23 "It looks like she's going to have a real good day," the willowy new aide with the easy smile tells Terry and me.

This is pleasant news, but I've never seen this aide before and I decide to give her a mini-introduction to Mom's water needs, as a precaution. "She can't get water for herself," I tell her. "She can't ask for it."

"Oh," she says, and her brow furrows; she looks slightly to the right of me. "She can't?" she says, the inflection telling me my tale is suspect.

"No. She'll die of thirst before she'll ask for a drink," I say, hoping to drive home the point with life-or-death drama. "Because she wouldn't know it—she wouldn't know that she was dying of thirst. You have to provide water within her reach. A small, clear glass is best. Sometimes it helps to prompt her." I'm not certain that she understands my meaning. "You know, point it out, physically offer it to her, that sort of thing."

"Okay," she says. "I will sure do that."

I am not as sure as she, but I believe she intends it. And I can understand her surprise and possible skepticism. If I could somehow hear them for the first time, my words might surprise me, too.

February 25   "Do you want to call anybody?" I ask Mom as we pass the phone in the hall. I'm thinking she will name Wayne or Sharon.

"Perry."

"Perry Como?"

"Yes."

"Hmm. I don't know his number. Do you?"

"No."

I roll her into the room. "How about we write him a letter?"

"Yes."

"That sounds good," Margaret adds from her recliner on the other side of the room.

I take out my notepad. "Dear Perry," I say aloud as I write the words. "Should I ask how he's doing?" Margaret and Mom agree this is a good idea. "Shall I tell him how much we like his songs?" Unanimous support again.

"Would you like to add something, Mom?" I extend the pad and pen toward her.

She takes the items from me, rolling the pen into the familiar grasp—How does this happen? Does the brain direct the hand, or do fingers themselves know this much of writing? She touches its point to the paper, makes a tight circle of ink below my writing. She studies the mark a moment, gazes off for a time—composing?—

then works again with the pen, careful and precise as an artist. She repeats this process several times, adding no visible word to the page, until the aides come to put her to bed.

"Are you finished?" I ask.

"No," she says.

The aides agree to come back shortly, then hurry off to other duties.

She looks up, then back down, writes some more. A small doodle. She hands the pen and paper back to me.

"Good work, Mom."

If only I could read her writing. Or her mind.

February 28 My mother's older brother Joe and his son decide to make the trip up from New Mexico to see Mom. Their arrival coincides with that of Sharon and her daughter on this last weekend of February. A feeling of last chance is in the air.

In contrast to our Christmas dinner broom closet experience, the seven of us share lunch in an almost elegant room, with carpeted floor, an oblong hardwood table, and a bank of windows running the length of two walls. An aide brings Mom's tray of typical nursing home fare, but serves her with a panache and air of respectful service that would do the finest restaurant proud.

Mom looks around the table, thronged by her family, smiles at each and is smiled upon. She is the silent center of attention, our *raison d'être*. She speaks only a handful of words during this hour together, but connects with each of us in her own way. Each relationship special—brother, nephew, granddaughter, daughters, son-in-law.

We understand that the seven of us will never gather again. I think Mom understands, too.

March 2 In preparation for moving out of this house at the end of the month—this house that we rented so that the three of us could live together—Wayne and I are excavating the closets this evening.

I pull out Mom's travel-scarred suitcase, open it to find the cast-off clothing of another incarnation of my parent. Garments my thrifty mother wore for years and years, every piece sewn and re-sewn and mended yet again: polyester pants with spent elastic; cotton blouses splashed with purple and lavender and rusty-red flower prints; her prosthetic bras, all-important only two years ago, forgotten now.

Fifty years of memories have unexpectedly been loosed. They wash over me now like a tsunami, and I am capsized.

As we drove up the mountain to our cabin this morning, our Subaru stuffed with our lives, Wayne and I got into an argument. A serious argument. About whether to keep or throw away a particular cardboard box. Argue—it's what we seem to do when we're afraid.

And now all these clothes, from which we can no longer hide. Mom gave them up long ago. And yet we save them, treasured tatters in a battered suitcase.

I don't want to live in this house anymore; would not have lived here at all but for the 644 days Mom was in it. We have no money to pay the rent anyway. We need to move. It's time.

Time also to let go of these old, no longer needed clothes.

34

Though much is taken, much abides; and though
We are not now that strength which in old days
Moved earth and heaven, that which we are, we are.
—Alfred Lord Tennyson,
"Ulysses"

March 4, Year Four   For thirty minutes I have visited with my mother-in-law—in her room, along the route to supper, here in the dining room. I've tried conversation, humor, and shtick. For the most part Mom has ignored me. She does not accept any help from me with her food. I decide she wants to be alone, and leave her to her dinner.

No sooner do I depart than Marilyn settles in next to her. I watch from the hallway as Mom smiles broadly, tilts her head toward her in greeting. Marilyn smiles, too, scoops a forkful of mashed potatoes from the plate and brings it to Mom's willing mouth. I feel a twinge of jealousy.

But I leave the building with something better: reassurance about moving farther away. As much as we love her and she loves us, this is her place. Maybe she'd like to have her own friends.

Maybe she already does.

March 10   This morning my mother is half asleep, trance-like. Sometimes she tries to talk to me, but even then her eyes do not open. I put oatmeal in her mouth. It remains there for a polite space of time, but finally the gruel succumbs to gravity and oozes out.

March 11 Mom has pneumonia. Terry tries to feed her breakfast in bed but she keeps falling asleep. I jiggle her legs and bounce on her mattress, anything to wake her up to take a little bite. Each time she does wake she smiles, and each smile tells me it's a whole new day for her.

Terry tells me that Kamilah told her that Mom is supposed to get her antibiotic by injection tonight. She tells me because this is not what she understood from the other nurse last night, and it is not what I understood, either. What we were told then was that the shot last night was a one-time injection, to be followed by oral antibiotics from then on.

I find Kamilah at the medicine cart and ask her if we can look at the order together. Terry and I are concerned, I tell her, because we had a different understanding. "I wonder if there could be an error of some sort," I say.

"You don't think that I am doing it correctly?"

The question rises to me from her beautiful brown face in slightly stilted phrasing and flavored with her sweet accent from a land I do not know. She is guileless, and not without feeling about my question.

"It's . . . just that I had understood it differently."

"I talked to the doctor," Kamilah says, and points to a note on the cart top. The name is my mother-in-law's. But her first name is spelled Hellen. "1mg i.m.," it says after her name, "then Biaxin."

She makes it clear that the doctor called today, that she talked to the doctor herself, and that this is a new order. The misspelling of Mom's first name seems in accord with what she tells me, that this is not yesterday's note but one which she has written herself today.

"Do they do that sometimes?" I ask. "Go back and forth from injection to oral, change the order?"

"Yes. And sometimes people get up to five shots on consecutive days."

I decide that the doctor is doing a doctor thing. Mom keeps getting sick, and she's trying to really knock out the infection this time. I am satisfied that Kamilah is doing exactly as she has been asked.

She readies the shot and I return to Mom's room, tell Terry that everything is as it should be. Marilyn comes in to turn Mom onto her side in preparation for the injection. Kamilah enters. We do not make eye contact.

* * * * *

Wayne is in search of food for us. Kamilah and Marilyn and I are with Mom. Kamilah has divided the large injection into two shots, one for each buttock. We make small talk, hoping that Mom can silently participate. We talk about eye color—the needle pierces Mom's skin, she flinches, Kamilah pushes the plunger slowly down —and point out each of our eye colors.

"I like brown eyes," Marilyn says.

Kamilah prepares the second shot, apologizes to Mom for having to give her these injections. "I don't want you not to like me," she says with a smile.

My mother looks up at Kamilah, who taps the syringe and sends a tiny arc of liquid through the air. She reaches up and places her hand on Kamilah's cheek, holds her there in her hand like a daughter. Like me.

"I love you," Kamilah says.

And I see that love, passing like grace itself between their dark brown eyes.

* * * * *

Terry tells me about Mom's and Kamilah's loving interaction. I want to say something to Kamilah, to undo, if I can, the stiffness that has developed between us.

"I think maybe you're a little angry at me," I tell her.

"Oh, no," she says and adds an apology if she caused me to think so.

"Oh, no," I say and apologize back. "It's not you, not anything personal. I do trust you. It's just that it was different than what I had understood, and different than what's been done before. It seemed possible that a mistake had been made. You weren't here last evening and I thought maybe you saw the order and didn't realize it had started last night. Somebody might have put the wrong date on it. Anything."

I don't recite the ten other possible scenarios that run through my mind; don't mention that I have seen errors made here before; don't remind her that there are dozens of sick people here, most of them receiving medications several times a day and that I understand that anybody could make an error—Kamilah, myself, anybody—that we're just trying to make sure Mom doesn't receive an incorrect dosage.

All of these things I don't say. And without my saying them, all of these things Kamilah understands.

"We love her very much . . ." I tell her, a small knot suddenly in my throat.

"Yes," she says firmly. "And it is your duty to take care of her, and watch out for her."

I am startled. She understands my position perfectly, is telling me that we would have been derelict not to have questioned her. "Yes," I say. "Exactly."

"We were both doing what's best for her."

"Yes," I agree again. I appreciate that she speaks so plainly, and that she understands—values, I think—who we are. "It might happen again sometime," I tell her. "I'll come up and say, 'What are you doing?' If that happens, it's because we want the best for her."

She nods. A comfortable nod that harbors no hard feelings.

Is there anything better than to be heard, to be known by another, and accepted still?

March 12 My mother eats only a little supper, and can't drink very well at all. Always a lover of the night sky, she says she wants to go look at the full moon when I offer to take her, but even from behind the safety of the day room windows she seems more frightened than awed.

And she is coughing. She can't stop.

Marilyn suggests the nebulizer and we put the mask on her. It scares her at first. "Mom," I tell her, "you don't have to go through all this if you don't want to. It's up to you what you want to do."

March 13 She lies there, a whimper on every exhale. I turn the oxygen-maker on, but struggle to get the tubing over her ear. I've seen Ryan and Kamilah do this a dozen times, always as quick and smooth as slipping on a pair of eyeglasses. But it's not that easy, it seems, not for me. I'm afraid I'll frighten her, hurt her even, with my clumsy attempts. I talk to her the whole time about what I'm trying to do. She offers no resistance, shows no pain or fear.

"I love you," I tell her. "Terry loves you. . . . We know you're not feeling good, and whatever you want to do, that's what we want for you. . . . Your body can't last forever. . . . We'll always love you, whether you're here with us in this body or not."

I hold her hand as I speak, and caress her head, combing with my fingers the silky, damp curls. Birds twitter and a stream gurgles from a CD in the background.

"I'm glad you came to live with us. I never expected that, never even thought about it happening ever. . . . We had some fights, you and I. You're not a grudge holder. Thanks for that."

Her whimpering has ceased. Birds, soft words, and affection fill the room. Marilyn passes down the hall. "Marilyn's here, Mom. And Kamilah. You're surrounded by love. . . . If there's any pain, just let go of that."

I repeat these themes, love and letting go, over and over, and all the while the room sweetens, like a spring morning with sun-drenched alyssum at the door. Mom's eyelids sag. Asleep, she clasps my hand in both of hers like a treasured doll.

"Now I'm going to take my hand out," I whisper softly. "Slowly . . . slowly." I repeat the words, wiggling my fingers, withdrawing, and after five minutes my hand is free. She sleeps still as I tiptoe into the bright wash of hallway lights.

March 15 At nine in the morning Mom is already being put to bed. "She's really not feeling well," the aide says, and she is right. Mom closes her eyes. Even in sleep, every breath comes hard.

March 16 She can't drink. We try feeding her. She can't eat. Wayne asks Ryan about an IV, blood work, an increase in her antibiotics. Anything.

Even in bed and asleep she looks really ill. But now she wakes, opens her eyes and smiles this incredibly angelic smile at me. For a moment it's completely wonderful, but the moment does not last. Soon her mouth drops open. Her eyes are wild and desperate.

Mom's doctor calls just past noon. "Her labs are horrible," she tells us. Her WBC is still high; her electrolytes are in terrible shape. She has given an order to start an IV. "It won't be an easy thing to get her system back in alignment at all," she warns. "Or in time." The electrolyte imbalance might cause any number of problems— heart arrhythmia, heart attack, convulsions—and certainly could be contributing to or be the underlying cause of her difficulties with swallowing. "Her little body," the doctor says, "is so weak . . ."

"We understand," we tell her.

And we understand, too, what she has not said.

— 35 —

To see a World in a Grain of Sand
And a Heaven in a Wild Flower
Hold Infinity in the palm of your hand
And Eternity in an hour
　　　　　　　　　—William Blake,
　　　　　　　　　　　"Auguries of Innocence"

March 17, Year Four　Her sleep exudes effort and focus, as though it consumes more energy than it returns. Despite the antibiotics, the IV, the full-time oxygen, Mom's body wants to sleep and do nothing else. Sleeping is as much as she can manage.

March 18　"I will tell you the new developments now," Kamilah says as soon as she sees me today.

She says that the doctor has discontinued the IV due to improvement of the latest blood results; that the needle remains in my mother-in-law's vein because she gets one more dose of antibiotics tonight through the IV; that there will be another blood draw in the morning, and an X-ray, too; that if all the results are satisfactory, she will disassemble all these tubes tomorrow.

I stay for many hours, setting up a laptop computer "office" for myself in her room. I work at my little desk—her feeding table, which I find to be more fun than working at my real desk—and as I work I glance out the door to the hall at all the familiar faces of the staff and residents passing by; look over my shoulder at Mom, too. So many times, we just look and smile.

Through the afternoon Kamilah tends to Mom and to Margaret, apologizing each time she enters. "You're not disturbing us," I tell her. The aides, too, are in and out with their duties. Sometimes I offer to help, but mostly they refuse. Mostly, it all goes on as if I'm not here. All this caring.

March 20   Mom's doctor calls to tell Wayne and me that she is amazed at how much better Mom is doing, that 70% of people with sodium levels as high as Mom's was, die. "She's doing better," she cautions, "but she's not out of the woods."

March 22   Whatever progress Mom has made has slipped away. "Cough that up," Ryan demands lightly. "You've gotta cough that up." Mom grins at him. "Oh, you think this is funny, huh?"

From all appearances, yes.

"I don't know where those smiles come from," he tells me.

I've never seen anybody this peaceful and loving. A person could say that her brain's deteriorated, that she's not burdened with worries and responsibilities, thoughts even, but I don't buy that totally. I think that some central part of my mother is revealing itself, coming to the fore with the assistance of this disease.

* * * * *

I talk with Ryan about Mom's ups and downs, how she's gone through this same pattern two weeks in a row and can't quite seem to break free of it, how I wish there was some way to get water into her more than half a teaspoon at a time.

He nods in agreement. "At that rate," he says, "you'd almost have to do it around the clock." He pinches the skin on the back of her hand, lets it go and watches the thin ridge of tissue stand for a second or two before slowly melting back into the veined landscape below. I watch, too, and do mental calculations of teaspoons and ounces. "She's kind of dehydrated," he says. And he's pretty much right in his "around the clock" estimate—getting half a gallon of liquid into her by half-teaspoon servings at one serving per minute would require twelve hours each day.

Ryan says he plans to keep her in bed for breakfast, then try getting her up for lunch, to see how that goes. I share this information with Terry.

"Unless they put her on an IV," Terry says.

"I asked about that. Ryan says the purpose of an IV is really to get her over a hump. I told him we've talked about that, you and I. That we understand that IV's can't be a way of life."

"No, but I'm not saying we shouldn't get another blood test. That'd be good. And if the test shows she needs it, we could do another IV."

"But like we said, she can't live on IVs."

"I know, but just to get her over the hump."

"We just did that. She was very hydrated. And now, three days later, she's dehydrated again."

"That's true. But she's still too weak to eat and drink enough on her own."

"That's what I mean. I think she's just too fatigued. Too worn out."

"I think we should do the blood test. And if it shows something, try the IV one more time."

March 23 Mom is weak and sleepy. I try to feed her when she wakes but she falls asleep again before I can get the food into her mouth. I call Terry. Any one of these slow deep breaths could be Mom's last.

She comes over with our neighbor Ella. Ella is shy and polite, but as an individual who has known and visited many sick and dying persons, as an elderly person herself, she has a view on what she sees here. While Terry visits at Mom's bedside, Ella gently tells me, "She's so tired. She needs to rest."

While the aide feeds Mom lunch, Terry and I talk on the phone with the doctor. "If we don't do anything, she's going to die," the doctor says. "I don't know how long it will take, but she will die." She has ordered another blood test, but she has called to see what we want to do. "It's up to you," she says.

"I don't know what to do," Terry says. "I don't have enough information. I don't feel like I know enough."

"I understand. But if I knew enough to know what will happen, what would be best for everybody, I'd be the greatest doctor."

There is silence on the line. I think the doctor is right. No one can know enough. Ever.

"Let's go ahead," Terry says. "Let's give it one more try."

March 24 This morning my mother cradles her teddy bear in her arm. She touches the dark nose gently, tugs lightly at her blanket as if to cover him.

She tries to talk. Though she doesn't say much anymore in words, her whole being speaks to me this very moment, tells me that she's pleased, that she's happy, that she's at peace. She is radiating love, like a great warming fire. I tell her, as I have for many weeks, that she is perfect just the way she is.

A friend told me recently, "Your mom is living with so much love. This might be the best time—the most blessed time—of her life." She could be right. I woke up this morning with this thought: the main thing is not what we decide to do. The main thing is the love.

I see her body, naked, see that the body of the woman who bore me is just skin stretched over bones. Her flesh is more desiccated than vital, too weak to bear her anywhere, too ethereal to hinder her. My mother is living now on smiles and love.

The best time of her life. If I am wise, this is the best time of my life, too.

Until now.

And now.

And now. . . .

* * * * *

My mother-in-law doesn't even flinch when the technician inserts the needle for the new IV. In a moment he has it taped down and her entire forearm wrapped in protective gauze.

"All done," I tell her as I move a strand of damp hair off her face. But it is not all done. Blood oozes around the insertion point. The IV is occluded. The tech takes it apart, removes the wrapping and the tape and the tubing and the needle. He searches her arm, squeezing and turning, tapping on veins that lie like blue threads beneath tissue paper skin, trying to find a route that will accept his medicine. When he does I pin Mom's innocent arm to the bed. "Here we go," he says, and pushes the needle in a second time.

Mom's arm kicks at the elbow and the tiny movement magnifies down the length of her arm, jerking her hand three inches. I can hardly believe what has happened; the suddenness, and the strength of her. Blood runs across her arm.

More searching and finally he finds yet another place, but this more difficult than either of the previous, because in order for him to insert the needle, Mom must hold her hand flat open.

Which she cannot do. Hold her hand open on request.

So he tucks his right elbow into the heel of her hand, then slides his elbow back, slowly, uncurling Mom's fingers as he goes, using his forearm as a restraint on her flattened palm. He readies the needle, which he holds also in this same right hand. It seems impossibly awkward. Again he needs me to hold her still. This time I take hold of her elbow with both hands, one above and one below, and weld it to the mattress with all the strength I have in me.

"Oh!" Mom yells as the needle pierces her.

Nothing moves.

"It's all right, Mom. Hold still." I feel her will flow down from her shoulder, feel her arm relax into a stillness of her own making.

Still holding the inserted needle in place with his right hand, still flattening her hand with his forearm, the tech reaches behind, finds his tape, fumbles with it one-handed, somehow gets a piece across the barrel of the needle and onto Mom's translucent skin. Then

another. And another. There is no bleeding. No oozing. No occlusion.
"You did really good, Mom. You did great."
"Yeah," the tech agrees, "you did really good."
Mom smiles at him, sharing in the victory. The outstretched fingers of her right hand caress his forearm, which rests still in the cradle of her palm, like that of an old friend.

March 26   Mom wakes from a deep sleep. She eats well in bed, has a good appetite. Wayne calls. I hold the phone to her ear and she listens, happy and relaxed.

"Guess what, Mom?" I say when she and Wayne are finished on the phone. "My birthday's coming pretty soon. Eleven days. You know what I'm going to do?" Her expression is pleasant, expectant. "I'm going to spend it with you!"

One more very big smile.

36

*[T]he nature of being is a constant erosion
of what is not essential.*

—Mark Nepo

March 27, Year Four   She is trying to talk, whole
sentences to me and the aide. We don't understand, but she doesn't
seem to mind. She is smiling. I think she's enjoying herself.

March 28   What a change from last night! Her mouth sags on the
right, and she looks exhausted.

I see fear in her, some kind of contraction—against dying?
pain?—and my first thought is, *Oh, Mom, don't be like that.* But no!
If she's feeling fear, she's feeling fear. She has a right to her feelings.
I want her to be exactly how she is.

I want to give my mother that more than anything, and I want
her to give that to me more than anything. That's what I want our
relationship to be. Acceptance.

April 1   At lunch we ask the staff to let my mother stay in her
room so that we can eat with her, but I don't know how they could
have gotten her up anyway. She looks too tired, too weak even to
lie in bed. Sometimes she looks right at me but nothing registers in
her eyes, as if I'm invisible. Other times she focuses intently, laser-
ing messages to me that I can't understand. She doesn't smile. Her
jaw is slack. She's breathing through her mouth even though she's
awake and has oxygen on.

I'm brimming with emotion, angry that she's worse on this very
day that Wayne and I are moving to our cabin eighty miles away.

Over and over I try to accept her as she is. Again and again I search for calm and an elusive peace.

Wayne moves close to her. "I guess we'll just have to love each other," he tells her. His words bring the only real smile I see on her face today.

April 2   In the twenty-four hours since we left town six phone messages have come to our Voice Mail, four of them about Mom. She isn't doing well.

It has snowed hard all day and as evening approaches the fat, wet flakes continue to fall—eight, nine, ten inches—covering us and our world in a cool and silent blanket of beauty. Terry and I can't go to Mom, but we believe that, like the quantum particles which compose our bodies, we can communicate at great distance instantaneously, and that once touched by another we remain forever connected. We talk to her where we are.

April 3   Wayne and I arrive at Meadowlark just past noon, after a two hour trip through fast-melting snow. I enter the room first and find Mom gulping for air. "Help me," her eyes say to me. "Do something."

I run to find Kamilah, who suggests the nebulizer. After a short treatment Mom falls asleep, and when she wakes ninety minutes later she looks entirely comfortable. They bring her food. She eats. Wayne juggles and pirouettes in her wheelchair to keep her awake between mouthfuls.

At 8:30 Kamilah is on duty. Lilith has joined her and will remain to also work her regular night shift. We feel comfortable leaving Mom in the hands of these two competent and caring women. We go to Christy and Zander's house for the night.

April 4   Four-thirty in the morning. My mother-in-law is sleeping heavily, breathing shallow, rapid-fire breaths, as though she's just finished a race. I watch the tiny heaves of her chest, count them against the clock: 38/minute, up from thirty last evening.

Lilith enters the darkened room, tells me that Mom had some distress around 2 a.m. She gave her a little water, a nebulizer treatment, and increased the oxygen flow. As far as she knows, she hasn't wakened since.

I sit quietly in the half dark, stroking Mom's leg, feeling the coolness of her knee against the palm of my hand with each pass. I contemplate this body before me which has been literally disappearing over the past year, perhaps both the result and a continuing exacerbation of her illness. Her physical self has melted away, cell by cell. Her intellectual and cognitive abilities have seemingly abandoned her. Yet she remains, becoming—with every passing day, with the departure of each molecule of flesh—an ever purer distillation of essential be-ing.

I hold her hand. It is warm and pliable, friendly, but does not grasp mine in return.

As difficult as coming to the nursing home has been from the beginning, I am aware that I have been coming for some months now more and more often, sometimes two or three visits in a single day. And I stay longer. Ostensibly, this is because of Mom's frailty, her need of Terry's or my hand to steady and maintain her delicate balance on the ever-thinning tightrope of her life. But the truth of the matter is that many times—this very morning—there is little to "do" once I get here.

No matter. More and more, we travel quiet paths. Someone who doesn't know us, glancing into this twilit room, might think it a sad sight—the middle-aged son with nothing to say to his dying mother. But the opposite is true: our communication has intensified. We no longer have much need of minds and mouths, of thoughts and words. More and more, it is our hearts that meet. More and more, our visits have become caresses.

* * * * *

I see that my mother has splotchy red marks around her knee. "Is that mottling?" I ask Ryan, thinking of the body's markings that presage death.

"Well, mottling does look just like that," he says, "but it usually starts from the toes up."

Her feet look normal, not dark or blotchy at all. She does look kind of dark, though. She is definitely dark in her face and neck.

Every now and then she takes a big, slow breath in her sleep. "You look so relaxed," I tell her. "That's the way it can be, Mom. Every day of our lives. No resistance. Let it come, let it go."

* * * * *

Her food just keeps coming in. We keep it for an hour each time. Just in case. Molly brings the evening meal now. "In one of my training classes we all picked someone we want to be like when we get old," she tells Terry and me. "I picked Helen."

"Thanks," Terry says. "For everything."

Molly steps out into the hall as if to leave, but her hand on the door jamb pulls her back. "Thank you," she says, "for being here."

I'm glad that I am here, too. And glad that Molly's here. Glad that we are all here. For a moment we are one person—Molly, Terry, Mom, and I, and all the world outside her door—made seamless by a shared flood of community and compassion.

It's 8:30 p.m. We haven't seen Mom's eyes since yesterday evening.

37

The world is but a bridge, build no house upon it.
Life is but an hour, spend it in devotion.
All the rest is the unseen.

—Akbar

April 5, Year Four The call comes in the middle of the night. Every cell in my body knows I cannot answer. I wrestle the phone off the night stand.

"Wayne," I say, and pass it to him beside me in the bed. He fumbles with the headset, hoists it clumsily to his cheek.

"Hello?" His voice is aged and deepened by sleep.

My fingers trace the cord that stretches across my chest in the silent dark.

It's Lilith. I know that.

"Okay," Wayne says after a few seconds. "We'll be right there." He hangs up, missing the cradle at first. "She said, 'Her breathing is barely moving.' I think she meant shallow. That her chest is barely moving."

It is 2:19 a.m. Actually 3:19, because of the Daylight Time transition just a few minutes ago. We dress without talking, move as efficiently and quickly as our numbed bodies and minds will allow. I glance again at the glow-red, impassive numerals: 2:29. What time is it really, I wonder, as we wend our way through the shadowy, familiar geography of our friends' house. It seems important to know.

Outside, the sharp night air jolts me fully awake and I leverage my tired body onto the seat of the International. In synchronous, mirrored motion we gird ourselves with flimsy grey belts, and pretend that we are safe, that Death will not overtake us. Wayne slips the selector into Drive. He doesn't speed, doesn't hurry overly much. His foot rests steady on the throttle.

At a red light he pauses just a moment, then swings smoothly through the left turn, no car in sight as far as the eye can see in any direction. The whole town is dark, sleeping.

Wayne pulls into the nearly empty lot. We slide off the high seat, walk quickly in determined silence across the asphalt, pass through the familiar heavy door. I hear its thud, already far behind us.

Everybody is in Mom's room it seems, churning along the length of her bed, busy under the harsh ceiling fluorescent. In truth there are only three staff, and the two aides leave as soon as we appear. Lilith finishes her work, spreads the smooth, white sheet smoother.

"She just died," she says quietly. "A few minutes ago."

My mother lies on her back, her mouth held closed by a rolled towel propped under her chin. A sweat covers her face like the lightest of veils. I bend and kiss her forehead, put my hands around her face and hug it to me. Forehead to forehead. She is still so warm.

"Damn," I tell her, "I miss you already."

Wayne plays "Bless This House" and follows it with "Ave Maria," Perry Como's rich, comforting baritone filling the room one last time. He takes Mom's left hand and my right. I clasp her right, and complete the circle. The warmth of her body seeps away.

* * * * *

My mother-in-law's body, long and straight, is arranged perfectly in the middle of the bed. Her face is pale and the skin is flabby, as though some padding she secretly carried there for eighty-one years has been removed.

A plain, white sheet covers her from the neck down, but I feel a strong and sudden need to see her. To see her whole body, head to toe. To assure myself that this is no magician's trick, that it is her, and that she is all here. That she is dead. That there is no mistake.

I lift the linen. Her legs are straight and lie flatter on the bed than they ever have since the day she fell. No more contractions. No more cough. No more choking. No more worry about how to get enough liquids into her. All of that is over. The sacred machine is irretrievably broken.

Her hands remain soft and pliable, but they have grown cooler now, and paler. Not white, like I might have imagined, but golden. Veins that I never noticed before have painted a map across the back of her hands and up her arms, and now pale from blue to lavender to orchid as I watch. The fingers, away from the veins, have turned progressively lighter but are fringed with a tremendous internal glow, as though tinted by a magnificent but hidden sunrise.

I am awed by the anatomy of a human being, its native beauty and elegance revealed to me in this body of Terry's mother. Vacated by spirit, no longer struggling to survive, I can better identify it now as a shell, a vehicle. A thing utilitarian and durable. Simple, yet complex beyond understanding. Noble.

In death, the body of this elderly woman—scarred, emaciated, exhausted though it is—looks to me neither frightening nor foreign, but familiar.

* * * * *

Ryan says he believes that people choose the time of their death. Says that he's gone in to people who have nobody to visit them, people who are unconscious, dying, and just hanging on and hanging on. He says to them, "All the people that you know have already been here and gone now. You don't have to wait anymore." And then, in an hour or two, they die.

I ask Lilith about Mom's last moments, what happened, how they unfolded. She says that she called us when Mom got "very shallow," and then again when she died shortly after, but we did not answer. She says that just before she died her respirations slowed dramatically. She more or less stopped breathing, I guess, and then took a very long deep breath. She did that three times—three breaths only—in the space of one minute. And then she didn't breathe anymore.

* * * * *

The fellow from the funeral home comes to retrieve the body. I hover nearby, a guardian. After he places it in the zippered cloth bag I tell him that I want him not to cover her face. He agrees, and I accompany him and the body down the corridor and out the front door. He places her in the vehicle, closes the door, and pulls away.

I return to Terry, and to Mom's forever-empty room.

— *Epilogue* —

"Be good to each other."

—Helen

April 6, Year Four I did not keep my promise to my mother. I am not spending my birthday with her as I said I would eleven days ago. But even in death she has kept a mother's implicit promise: she has birthed me again on this my anniversary day. Birthed me into mid-life, into a life all my own, a life happier and richer for having known her.

April 7 Wayne says that he's been walking around with a special feeling inside of him these last couple of days, despite the pain and sadness. "I feel like I'm brimming over, getting larger and lighter, like a balloon rising into the sky. Rising not by any effort, but by its pure nature," he tells me. "It isn't exactly happiness I'm feeling. More like joy, and wonder at life's sheer and unrelenting beauty."

We've been back several times to empty Mom's room. A single rose lies on her bed, a farewell, we think, from the staff. Everyone expresses their condolences. People hug me, allow my tears or cry with me. They treat us as though we are special. It won't go on forever, but I wish it would.

I think we should always be that way with each other. Everyone's had losses. Everyone has current and past griefs. For the twenty years after the death of my father until she came to live with us, my mother closed every audiotape letter she sent to Wayne and me with the words "Be good to each other."

Everyone deserves that much. All the time.

April 9 It is a mild spring day, but here inside the crematorium it is already hot. Wayne asks the undertaker to open the cardboard box. His request surprises me and I take an instinctive step back. "You look first," I tell him. "Tell me if it's okay." He says it is, and I look. The beauty of her face, the peacefulness, shocks me. There is no makeup. She hasn't been embalmed. It's just her.

We sit outside for a few minutes at a wrought iron table, provided, I suppose, for mourners. But I am not mourning. Somewhere behind and above me the *whirrr* of the crematory exhaust fan tells me that even now it is sending molecules of my mother into my lungs. I have heard it said that in my lifetime I will inhale an atom that was once a part of the body of Jesus Christ. If this is so, I suppose I breathe equally of Confucius and Abraham, Mohammed and Buddha and Lao Tsu. And of their children, and spouses, and neighbors, whose names the world has forgotten. In some far-distant future perhaps everyone on earth will breathe an atom of my mother. Everyone breathes everyone.

My mother once told me that she hoped she would die of a heart attack, quickly. She didn't. She died from Alzheimer's, slowly. Yet through those years she never stopped reaching out to life. We did not lose each other in the labyrinth of her disease. We found each other, in a new territory, one which lies beyond the horizons of personality and history and, finally, beyond the map of Mother-Daughter. A deep, essential place, where love is the only employment, the only medium of exchange, the only language.

I know that my mother's illness brought her losses. I believe that it brought her gifts as well, as I know it did to Wayne and me. In caring for her and being cared for by her, in loving her and being loved by her, she was our blessing, although a fierce one, which we hope we will be wise enough and brave enough to carry forward.

Hand in hand, we stroll across the street to a bakery, inviting Mom to join us for a pastry adorned with blueberries, strawberries, raspberries and kiwi. "Ah, wouldn't you know?" Wayne says wistfully as we settle at the little table. "They haven't even set a place for her."

ABOUT THE AUTHORS

Wayne Baltz is the co-author of four children's novels. He holds a BS in Education and an MS in Counseling Psychology, has taught in the public schools, worked with children and adults in psychiatric treatment settings, and administered an independent-living program for developmentally disabled adults. He has been presenting programs in schools since 1993.

Terry Baltz is the author of four picture books and the co-author of four children's novels. She co-authored a weekly newspaper column for children. She holds a BA in English and an MS in Human Development and Family Studies and is the primary author of a journal article on nursing home aide selection, published in *The Gerontologist*. She has coordinated parent education programs and taught developmentally disabled adults. She has been presenting programs in schools since 1993.

Terry and Wayne live in the Rocky Mountains of Colorado. Their nearest neighbors are deer and elk, badgers and bears, coyotes and bobcats, and incredibly starry skies.

The authors are available for interviews and to speak to professional, educational, and service organizations, employee groups, book clubs, and the general public. For further information, or to order books, visit them on the Web at www.fierceblessing.com or call 888-288-4841.